Deleting Diabetes
I did it. You can, too.

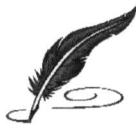

Joseph A. Onesta

www.mindpowerpittsburgh.com

ISBN: 978-1-7361870-5-0

Integrity HPI

Human Performance Improvement

www.integrityhpi.com

To contact the author, visit www.mindpowerpittsburgh.com

You should read this book!

If you or someone you love has type 2 diabetes, even if it is well controlled with medications, the information contained in these pages is for you. If you or someone you know has prediabetes, fatty liver disease, or metabolic disease, you are likely to benefit from this book. If you have dieted off and on, have tried fad diets, have lost and regained weight, this book can be life changing.

Traditional medicine is quite skilled at treating the symptoms of metabolic disease but often fails to address the central cause. Type 2 diabetes is just one symptom of metabolic disease. While traditional medicine is quite skilled at treating the symptoms of metabolic disease, we can address the fundamental cause of the disease itself.

Deleting diabetes as well as the other symptomatic conditions of metabolic disease, such as obesity, insulin resistance, cardiovascular issues, high blood pressure, digestive disorders, cancer, and even Alzheimer's, can be helped and, in many cases, reversed by a simple lifestyle change that fundamentally addresses the *cause* of metabolic disease.

Best of all, these conditions are not your fault. These conditions are not the result of a lack of discipline, willpower, or even lack of exercise. You have likely done what you have been told to do, *for the most part.* After all, no one is perfect. Now you have the opportunity to learn about simple changes that can make a world of difference. It's time to get your life back!

Table of Contents

Preface:
A Note to You from the Author

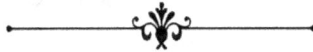

I want to be upfront with you. I intend to challenge you. Whether you accept my story at face value or place more or less stock in it is not my primary concern. I want to challenge you to embrace taking ownership and responsibility for your health and wellness. By that, I do not mean I want you to abandon the advice of your doctors. They know more than most of us, and frankly, we need them. But we also need to understand what their advice means and entails.

When I was just a kid, doctors were saints on earth. They made house calls, cultivated amazing bedside manners, checked on the sick regularly, answered the phone in the middle of the night, and in general, inspired confidence. I do not think many doctors are like that today. Although, I suspect that many of them wish they could be.

When I was five years old, I took a hard fall when letting go of a swing. Landing on my behind, I got up and continued playing. After all, I was just a kid, and kids fall a lot. The next day I was in such pain that I could not walk. When my parents tried to lift me, I screamed. They rushed me to the emergency room. At that moment, our family doctor was walking through the emergency room and saw me. "Get this child to Children's Hospital now." My parents did so, and I spent weeks in traction and then weeks in recovery at home to the point I had to learn to walk again.

That story became part of our family history, extolling the wisdom of that doctor, but what was the real wisdom he displayed? I was in a hospital at the time. Could he not have cared for me there? The truth was, he couldn't care for me at all, and he knew I would be better served at another hospital that specialized in the needs of children under the care of a doctor who focused their practice on children.

Today we have specialists for every medical concentration. The extent of medical knowledge has grown exponentially in the last fifty years. We cannot possibly expect our family physicians to know and apply it all. According to an article by Peter Densen, MD, titled "Challenges and Opportunities Facing Medical Education," in the *National Center for Biotechnology Information (NCBI)*, in 1950, it would take an expected 50 years for medical knowledge to double. When the article was written in 2011, it was anticipated that medical knowledge would double at a rate of every 73 days by 2020—*doubling* every 73 days! How is anyone expected to keep up? It is no wonder doctors do not have time to make house calls anymore.

Indeed, I wonder if even specialists can keep up in their areas of expertise. How many of us have sought a second and third opinion on a diagnosis, prognosis, or recommended course of treatment only to end up with a confusing choice?

The information age presents us with the unique challenge of misinformation but also provides us the opportunity to investigate, research, learn and make more informed decisions than ever before. I believe we are very quickly entering an age where we need to do just that, and if we do not, we are taking a big gamble.

My first step toward that specific goal happened a number of years ago when my doctor wanted to prescribe a third diabetes medication to postpone injecting insulin to gain control of my blood glucose levels. To me, injecting insulin represented a point where the probable outcomes became inevitable. I asked him to present me with options so I could read about them. Before that moment, I would have accepted anything he said as truth and gospel. Something inside me compelled me to stand up inside, be brave, and know that I needed to understand what was going on in my body and life.

My story is, I believe, a good one, but it is just that, my story. I hope you enjoy it, and I dare to hope you find it inspiring. However, my story adds no more than another example of anecdotal evidence for the metabolic science to which I ascribe.

I knew very little when I began my quest. I didn't even know the difference between type 1 and 2 diabetes. I didn't understand what my medications were intended to do in my body. I certainly didn't have the slightest glimmer of understanding of why diabetes had singled me out as a victim.

I had a lot to learn, and just like good science, there's always more and more. Science is evolving. Our understanding grows and changes with new information. What science seems to prove is just an indication of further questions that need to be answered. I'll never know it all, neither will you. Not even your doctor would claim to know it all and if they do, find a new doctor. Certainly, they know more than you do, but their knowledge has stopped growing if they have stopped asking questions. Such a condition is not a sign of a good scientist.

As for me, it was only through research, soul-searching, and a certain degree of biohacking (self-experimentation) that I was able to delete diabetes. I have not taken diabetes medications for years, and my A1C, a three-month average of blood glucose levels, has been 5.4 or less throughout that time. I've taken insulin resistance tests twice and have been rated as insulin sensitive. For all intents and purposes, one might assume that all traces of diabetes are gone from my life, that I am effectively cured of the disease. I am hesitant to suggest that.

When we delete something from our computer, the file is not obliterated. It simply is no longer referenced, and that part of the computer's memory is marked as available for overwriting. It is in that sense that I have deleted diabetes. Whether or not those original files have been overwritten or whether or not they will ever be overwritten is a question to ponder but seems to be unanswerable at present.

I don't know if my files have been overwritten or not, but one thing I do know is that if I go back to living and eating the way I had been when I developed the condition, I suspect that diabetes could easily return. If you take anything from this book beyond encouragement, know that if you choose to delete your diabetes, the changes you make to do that most likely need to be permanent.

I also think it is fair to tell you that the changes are not the easiest ones to make. It's been my experience that those changes get easier as we go, but it is easy to fall back into old patterns. Whenever we make fundamental changes in our lives, our bodies and minds have to battle their way through. For me, being diabetes-free is that peace won after a brutal war. If it weren't for the help of hypnotist colleagues, my own practice of self-hypnosis, and mindfulness, the change would have been much more difficult. For that reason, I've included a self-hypnosis book in my suggested reading list.

About my challenge for you, I am reminded of one of the stories I use in my hypnosis practice. I'll summarize it here because it illustrates the kind of change necessary to delete diabetes successfully.

Jerrod was twelve years old and was on his first Boy Scout camping trip. Several troops were camping together on this outing, and the scout leaders had constructed an obstacle course out of a playground in the middle of the campgrounds. Each scout leader monitored an obstacle, and each troop was timed at each obstacle with a calculation applied to account for some troops having more scouts than others.

One of the obstacles was a set of monkey bars. Being on

the chubby side, Jerrod could never really do well at monkey bars. He'd lose his grip on the second or third rung and fall to the ground. He watched in horror as a boy from another troop dropped down from the bars as Jerrod knew he would. The scout leader blew his whistle and made the boy try again. Three times, the boy was forced to try again; all the while, the clock was ticking. Jerrod felt his shame and humiliation and knew it would soon be his own.

Something happened in Jerrod's mind as he approached the monkey bars. A crazy idea came to him. He thought he might see his way through this problem. It probably would not work, but it was worth a try. So, instead of reaching for the cross rung and trying to swing rung to rung, he used all his strength to hoist himself up on top of the monkey bars. He then crawled across the obstacle, waiting for the scout leader to blow his whistle.

There was a bit of chatter from the other troops, but the whistle never came, and Jerrod proceeded onto the next obstacle with his fellow troop mates.

You see, sometimes we think there is only one right way of doing something. If we can't manage it in the traditional way, we are doomed to the consequences. A doctor says you have diabetes and calls in a prescription to your pharmacy. Most don't question it at all, and we keep trying, going along the best we can. We work our way through increased dosages, new medications, additional medications, and even several types of insulin.

Watching that A1c rise is like falling off the monkey bars. Contrast Jerrod with the other boy who dropped from the monkey bars three times and had his speed significantly penalized by the repetition. Eventually, both boys went on but to what end? Which boy left that competition with fewer emotional scars and with more confidence?

Will you just go on trying again and again like that first boy doing the same thing over and over again only to get the same result, or will you, like Jerrod, climb up on top of the monkey bars? Will you simply accept the prognosis of "chronic and progressive," or will you be like others who have chosen to find a different way? The decision is yours, and whether you take up my challenge or simply stay the same, it is a decision you will own and for which you will be responsible.

Chapter 1:
The Dreaded D-Word

❧

❝The doctor says you're diabetic, so watch what you eat," That's exactly what the office assistant said to me. The words are seared into my memory. I believe I can still hear her voice! She said it offhand, just like that, almost flippantly.

I was stunned, almost speechless. Whatever I expected, it wasn't that. All I could say was, "What do you mean? Watch what I eat?"

"I don't know. They have classes over at the hospital." I could hear her chewing gum. "I can give you the number."

"Can I please speak with the doctor?"

"She isn't here. Do you want the number?"

I hung up on her. It was partly the shock. I was angry, confused, and frankly incredulous. Was I supposed to take such news casually? Should I have just thanked the office assistant for the heads-up and been on my merry way taking notes about what I was eating? How did diabetes happen to me? Why wasn't my doctor making that call? Wouldn't she expect me to have questions that an office assistant could not answer?

That was back in the fall of 2004. We had just moved from Long Beach, California, back to my hometown of Pittsburgh, PA. My father had just passed away, and like many other people my age, I returned to my hometown to be with my family and, most importantly, my 84-year-old mother.

I decided to write the doctor a letter explaining what happened and my reaction to it. I asked her to call me at her convenience. If she preferred that I see her with an appointment, I'd be glad to make one, but I just had a few questions.

A month passed by with no response to my letter, so I decided to find another doctor. I called the office and ordered a copy of my medical record, for which I had to pay $20. I picked up the hefty file, went through it, and discovered my letter was not included. I could only guess that either the doctor never got the letter or, more likely, she never saw it. I could just imagine that office assistant slipping it into the shredding machine. What was done was done.

I'll confess I wasn't too keen on finding another doctor right away. Was it denial or avoidance? Probably it was a bit of both, but then life took a turn. My insurance had run out, and I had started a new consulting job that required extensive travel. I'd leave my home on Sunday evenings and return Friday afternoons. Scheduling appointments was difficult, and I wanted to be well established in the job before I started requesting days off. All totaled, I quit that job after six months, and it was nearly a year before I would again meet a doctor for a physical.

When I finally found a new doctor, I hoped against all hope that he wouldn't use the D-word. Well, I experienced my existential comeuppance. The diagnosis was the same. This time, I got the news in person; no office assistant gave me the diagnosis, no gum chewing in my ear. He took time to explain to me what it meant to have diabetes, that it was a chronic and progressive illness, but it could be managed with medications, diet, and exercise. He gave me a prescription for metformin, said he wanted to see me again in six months, and referred me to a nutritionist/dietitian.

My doctor said that I suffered from a condition known as metabolic syndrome. In medicine, calling something a syndrome means that they do not know where it comes from. Genetics may play a part, but they just do not know. He said I had fatty liver disease, which I did not understand except for the word fatty. Well, we knew why I was fat, didn't we? I overate and didn't exercise enough, right? It was a very oblique way of suggesting it, my being fat, and consequently, my diabetes, was somehow my fault, at least in part.

As I left his office, a wrestling match was going on in my head. For the first time in my life, my mortality was made real to me in more than an intellectual way. It is one thing to know that death comes to us all and another thing entirely to be told how I was going to die. He didn't say those words, but what other interpretation is there for diabetes?

Diabetes was uncommon in my family and had been rare in my life experience. Diabetes wasn't something I really understood or had even considered, at least not for me. I had a friend whose husband, Lenny, was severely diabetic. He was often hospitalized and, starting at the toes, began to require amputation until he had lost his legs entirely and eventually died. That was the picture I had in my head as I processed the information my doctor provided.

For the first time in my life, I thought I knew how I would die. I had a prescription for pills and an appointment with someone who would tell me how to control the sugar monster inside me. There was no cure; the disease would progress, and I would end up like Lenny, rotting from the inside out, having bits and pieces cut off, and perhaps going blind until there remained too little of me to hold onto life.

Until the diagnosis, only one thing in my life had ever been permanent. In the sixth grade, I had accidentally stuck myself in the leg with a pencil. After she cleaned my wound, the school nurse told me the mark left under my skin by the graphite would be there forever. Forever! It's still there, and I sometimes look at it just to see.

The permanence scared me. It had taken years for me to pierce my ear even though "everyone" was doing it. I have never really ever considered a tattoo. When I bought my first car, my first house, and when I decided to move across the country, I had to talk myself into it by assuring myself that I could always change my mind. I could sell or move back. The graphite under my skin was my first experience of an existential crisis.

The nutritionist was exceptionally nice, patient, compassionate, and genial. We met in a little room fitted out like a break room with a table and chairs. We sat next to one another instead of across a desk. She told me that lots of people lead happy, healthy lives with diabetes, and she was going to show me how to live the best I could.

She gave me a diagram of the food pyramid. I had seen it before. I walked away from that meeting with relatively simple ground rules, most of which I had already been following. I'll tell you about that later. There were, however, some notable differences. She recommended that I eat up to 60% of my daily calories from whole-grain carbohydrates. I hadn't thought about whole grain products. Of course, the idea that whole grains were a healthier choice had reached my awareness but wasn't something I had considered much before.

The most significant shift for me was her suggestion to eat smaller, more frequent meals, basically, snacks, to keep my blood sugar levels stable. I could certainly do that. It meant a bit more planning. Snacks were easy to find, but whole grain snacks were harder to come by.

She also suggested I increase my exercise, which was something I was eager to do now that traveling for work was out of the equation. Back in California, I swam laps three or four times a week. I'm a good swimmer. I love to swim. Finding a pool in Pittsburgh, however, was not easy.

Eventually, I found a gym with a pool but soon realized

I had wasted my money. People were just bobbing around in the pools with very few lanes reserved for swimming laps. Those lanes were always occupied. I hate sharing lanes. Other swimmers are usually slower or much faster than me. Two people sharing a lane is okay if we agree to split the lane in half. The moment a third person joined, dividing the lane was over.

It sounds like I'm making excuses, I know. I tried. Swimming in Pittsburgh was nothing short of aggravating. Sometimes I'd get in a few laps, but soon there would be that third person. We'd have to swim in circles, and that third person invariably wanted to do the breaststroke. It was just too slow for me. I love swimming, but I hated swimming in Pittsburgh. I tried to find a pool where you could reserve a lane, but it was not to be. Of course, I did other things at the gym, but I didn't really enjoy them, and not bothering to go at all became easier and easier.

There was nothing unusual about the advice I was given. It was, and often still is pretty standard advice. I followed the advice almost religiously. I say almost because everyone wavers once in a while. Whole grains dominated my pantry, although I refused to compromise on whole wheat pasta. I found it disgusting and figured that if everything else were by the book except for a plate of spaghetti once in a while, I'd be alright. I even made cakes out of whole wheat flour.

Everything went along steadily, and the metformin seemed to be doing the job. Ten years in, I gave up added sugar for a whole year. The only sweet I allowed myself was whole fruit, fresh or dried. There was no candy, cakes, or cookies—nothing with added sugar. I even cleaned out my pantry of food that listed added sugars in the ingredients.

I'm going into this detail because I want you to know I was a reasonably good type 2 diabetic doing precisely what the doctor and the nutritionist advised me to do. I wasn't always perfect and, I suppose, neither are you, or you wouldn't be reading this book. Their advice was the industry standard. They told me to do what they had been taught to tell type 2 diabetics. I had no reason to question it.

However, there is a problem with that advice. In terms of stabilizing blood glucose levels, along with medications, the advice isn't bad. The problem is that the advice assumes that type 2 diabetes is both chronic and progressive. It assumes that the best we who have been diagnosed with type 2 diabetes can hope for is to slow down the inevitable progression of the disease by controlling blood sugar levels through medications. I no longer accept those assumptions as facts. I have joined the thousands of people who have demonstrated that the assumptions are wrong.

I hope you are interested in learning and doing what thousands of diabetics are doing to not only control but actually reverse the progression of type 2 diabetes and potentially delete it from your life. Imagine turning the whole thing around. What if your blood glucose levels could be in the normal range, not even prediabetic? Imagine your doctor cutting the dosage and perhaps even eliminating your diabetes medications. You could have more energy, stamina, and be more alert. You can eat until you are satisfied. You can banish cravings and all but the most honest hunger pangs. You will find yourself enjoying life more. Imagine excess body fat melting away. When that happens, you get a whole new wardrobe!

Chapter 2:
How Diabetes Happened to Me

W hen I asked my doctor how I had acquired type 2
diabetes, he couldn't really say. He explained that I
suffered from a condition called metabolic syndrome. The
condition was indicated because a blood test specified fatty
liver disease and elevated blood glucose levels. His
explanation sufficed at the time, but that begged the question
in my mind: *How did I get the metabolic syndrome?*

That's just it, you see. If the medical profession calls a
condition a syndrome, it means that they don't really know
where it comes from. They might suspect a genetic
predisposition, but the cause has not been definitively
determined. I believe that we do know the cause of metabolic
disease. I also have a good guess at why it is still often called

a syndrome. I will give you my explanations in the next chapter. But first, let me tell you about my experience. I wonder how many things we have in common.

When I was a kid, having a stay-at-home mom was normal. Most kids had stay-at-home moms. The term "latchkey kids" first appeared during WWII when dads were off fighting and moms were pulled into the workforce. Kids might go home and take care of themselves for a few hours until mom got home. After the war, the term went out of vogue until it became an issue in the 1980s. For economic reasons and somewhat because women's roles in society were changing, latchkey kids became more common.

My mother, though trained and licensed as a beautician (the old name for cosmetologist), did not work outside our home apart from the occasional haircut for a relative or friend. She was always there when I got home from school, usually standing at the stove stirring something. When my father walked through the door after work, it was dinner time. We sat around the table together, all at the same time, and we all ate what she cooked.

My father worked a physically demanding blue-collar job in a steel mill. The meals my mother prepared were what she called balanced. They were hardy and filling and centered on protein, in other words, meat. There were one or two vegetables and a small portion of what my mother called "starch," usually potato, pasta, or a slice of homemade bread. Everything was homemade. There was no dessert. We ended the meal with salad, and there were no store-bought dressings. We rarely, if ever, ate in restaurants. My mother bought no prepackaged food other than breakfast cereal. The only carb-heavy meal we ate happened on Sundays. It was an early meal of pasta, meat, and salad. If we had a dessert, it happened on Sunday.

Going out for treats was even rarer. I remember one time and one time only when my father bought me an ice cream cone. It was just the two of us. There were probably more occasions, but I don't remember them. I was about 10 years old. On that particular day, my father took me to his work under the pretense of going to his credit union. We went into the place he called the boiler room. The room was dark. Men walked around in asbestos suits among huge crucibles filled with molten steel. Sparks and glowing lava, the place fulfilled every image of hell I had ever contrived.

I must have been visibly shaken because my father took me to a local soft-serve ice cream stand. Sitting in the car, licking, trying to keep ahead of the melting soft serve, he sprung the trap.

"If you don't do well at school and go to college, that is where you are going to work."

Enough said. I knew I was going to college no matter what.

As first-generation Italian Americans who had lived through not only the war but the Depression as well, my parents were sticklers for the highest quality at the best price. In those days, quality wasn't all that hard to come by, even in the supermarket. Many fresh foods were still seasonal. There was no GMO (genetically modified organisms) anything, and if people bought baked goods at all, they bought them from a bakery or an old-fashioned bake sale.

In Pittsburgh, we have a shopping district called The Strip District. The Strip was a kind of distribution hub for rail and trucking companies. Primarily warehouses and wholesale dealers, a few stores were open to the public where the freshest and highest quality products, many of them imported from Italy, could be purchased.

My parents would come home with entire wheels of cheeses, yards of sausage and pepperoni, and those special ingredients from the old country that most supermarkets did not even know about back then. Because they grew up during the Depression, they were into stockpiling food.

Our garage housed a huge chest freezer filled with meat and poultry, bought, slaughtered, and packaged on a farm in nearby Ohio where one could contract for half a cow. If you purchased the whole cow, it was even cheaper. So, my folks usually went in on a whole cow, a pig, and chickens with other relatives. Throughout the year, every few weeks, there'd be a drive back to Ohio, only about 30 miles away, for farm-fresh eggs. Every summer, my father planted a large garden and sometimes bought bushels of vegetables at roadside stands. There would be whole days spent canning and freezing that produce, which lasted through the winter.

Today, such products and produce come at a premium, sometimes outrageous, prices, but for us, fresh, high-quality food was normal.

Processed or packaged foods were uncommon in our house, but they were also comparatively uncommon in the market. Such things weren't part of our shopping list. My mother often made our bread, pizza, and pasta at home.

Products like potato chips, ice cream, or candy were rare treats. Cake, always homemade, was for birthdays. Cookies were for holidays, graduation parties, and weddings. The very idea of a snack carried the connotation of "treat." Treats didn't come every day. For a treat to be a treat, it was rare and special. I remember being jealous of other kids whose mothers gave them bags of chips or packaged cookies or cakes in their lunches. Of course, I wanted such things. I was a kid. My bag lunches included a sandwich and a piece of fruit. We bought milk at school.

I had toys, but my play life didn't revolve around them, even in the winter when there was sledding, snowball fights, and snowmen to build. In the summers, I played outside all day. The neighbors had a pool. We made up games and played at the neighborhood schoolyard. We didn't have a park, but we had woods, and there too, we got up to all sorts of fun and, I confess, a bit of mischief.

Perhaps I'm over-sentimentalizing my youth, but life was truly very different then. I admit I occasionally nabbed a meatball while my mother was frying them or covered a slice of homemade bread with some pasta sauce in anticipation of the meal, but snacking wasn't part of what we did. Our fridge always held cured meats, cheeses, olives, and pickled vegetables. If one was hungry and a meal wasn't in the offing, there was something to eat.

By the time I was 10, I could slice bread and cook my own breakfast, "cook" being the operative word. We had cereal, but it was never the sugary kind that a kid wanted. Young people rarely learn to cook anything unless they have designs on culinary school. Families rarely eat together except perhaps out of a greasy bag on the way to soccer practice. Both parents have to work, so freezers are filled with things that can be heated in the microwave or the toaster oven. I doubt most kids today could identify butcher paper if they saw it. And the vast majority would not be trusted with a bread knife.

I grew up eating healthy, good quality, real food.

I graduated high school in 1978. I was considered a bit overweight compared to the other boys my age. Most boys in my graduating class had a waist size of 28 or 30 inches. My waist was 34. I was in the school band and had fairly thick thighs from marching. Levi's 501 jeans, the ones with the button fly, were popular back then. I couldn't get them over my thighs despite the waist being my size or even a size bigger. I wore the 560s, which had a loose leg fit.

I felt fat, thought I was fat, and in my teenage angst, hated being fat. In retrospect, I wasn't really fat, but simply not thin, and there is a big difference. I was a big guy and could well have played football or rugby if I had been so inclined. I wanted to be skinny, wished I could fit into a size medium shirt, and wear 501 jeans. In my class of more than 250 people, only a few students, perhaps three, would be considered obese today. That's little more than 1% of the student body. Today, kids their size are quite common, if not the majority.

Things changed drastically when I went to college, where I was free to eat whatever I wanted as long as I could afford it. I couldn't afford to eat the way I did at home. My diet significantly changed in college, partly because I got to eat what I wanted, and I was little more than a kid. I liked that freedom and was given to indulge occasionally in the products I rarely, if ever, got at home. Additionally, the quality of the food available wasn't the same standard as my parents demanded. Few people could hold a candle to my mother in the kitchen.

I had only about $20 a week to spend on food and other expenses. I lived in a house with a bunch of other guys. It was a religious group. We prayed in the morning and ate breakfast together five days a week. Keep in mind we were students. Everything was on a budget, and most of what we ate was pretty simple to cook. Not all of the guys were useless in the kitchen, and we didn't spend our budget on pizza and buckets of fried chicken, but we did buy the cheapest groceries we could get for the things we knew how to cook. We made our own version of McDonald's breakfasts. We bought eggs, English muffins, cheese, and frozen hash browns. Those group meals pretty much took up a fair portion of my budget.

To eat and for a little extra money, I worked a few hours a week in the cafeteria, which meant I could go into the dining room anytime I liked, whether I was scheduled to work or not. No one knew the difference. Once inside, I could eat. I wasn't the only one doing that. I struggled with the dishonesty of it, but I also saw how much food my fellow students wasted. At least I was eating it.

If one ate what the cooks had planned, it was better balanced than the food I got in the house with the guys. As I have already indicated, I didn't always make the best choices.

In any case, even the cafeteria menu was constructed out of the cheapest ingredients they could get, just like restaurants. There was a kind of meat product that came in a long plastic tube, and I shudder to think what kind of meat was in it. At best, it was a giant hotdog that the cooks sliced into portions and covered with gravy made out of a powdery mix. Everything on the menu was mass-produced. There were bags of frozen French fries or powdered potatoes and massive cans of vegetables, all heated in huge vats. The only fresh food was found on a kind of salad bar half stocked with canned pudding and Jello.

I went into grad school almost directly from undergrad. My living situation had changed. I shared a ramshackle trailer with a roommate. Rent was cheaper, but my food budget was even more dire. I lived on rice, pasta, and generic mac and cheese. Meat came in the form of cheap hotdogs and breaded veal patties, glove-shaped meat products that came four for a dollar. I remember once finding 17 cents in a parking lot and thinking, *Great, I can get an onion for my rice!* I was cooking for myself, but I couldn't afford food that wasn't dirt cheap. Poverty comes at a nutritional price. What is cheap is often not healthy.

By 1986, I had a master's degree and a 38-inch waist. I'm convinced that the only reason I wasn't fatter was because a fair portion of the time, I did not eat and because I didn't have a car, I had to walk everywhere. I moved to New York City and began teaching at several branches of City University. I spent a lot of time on campus working with my students and a lot of time on the subway getting from one campus to another.

My apartment in the Bronx was a 40-minute subway commute if the trains were running properly. My neighborhood was pretty nice. I lived near the junction of Jerome Avenue and Gunhill Road. There was a business district with bodegas, a grocery store, a bagel store, a deli, a diner, and several take-out food vendors.

However, I was living alone for the first time in my life. Eating was still a problem. Though I had learned from my mother how to cook many things, I rarely cooked a meal unless I was having guests, and often, we would simply go out to eat. More often than not, I just picked up something to take home.

I spent most of the day too busy to eat a real meal. I'd grab a bagel and coffee on my way to the subway. I'd get an order of fries or a slice of pizza between classes as I traveled to another campus. By the time I was headed home, I was very hungry and too tired to cook. I'd get take-out. It might be Chinese, Indian, fast food, Chino-Latino, Greek, a deli sandwich, or even a quick pass through one of the ubiquitous greengrocer salad bars that dotted the city. My default was a take-out place on my corner that sold half a fried chicken with a big side of fries for $5. After college, believe it or not, spending a whole $5 on a meal felt like a splurge.

Because I had grabbed nibbles on the run, in my mind, I hadn't really eaten all day. Because I was eating mostly carbohydrates, I felt hungry all the time. I learned firsthand that carbohydrates create their own kind of hunger, but when you're on the run, you get what is fast and convenient. You don't feel like you have much choice.

Throughout the city, one could get a large slice of pizza for a dollar. If you wanted something other than cheese, you had to wait or hope they had it handy. I never had time to wait. By the time I was headed home, I was exhausted and felt like I was starving. My eyes were often bigger than my stomach, and I nearly always bought more than I should have. A half chicken and fries are, or should be, enough food for two, not one. Being a card-carrying member of the clean plate club, I ate until the food was gone in a single meal.

When I moved to Japan, where City University had a branch campus, I still didn't cook much, but eating out in Japan was different from New York. The portions were much smaller and set menu meals made eating a more balanced diet easier. Most restaurants had display cases of plastic replicas of meal options on the menu. Before I could speak enough Japanese, all I had to do was point.

Near my apartment on campus was a noodle shop, which served up salty bowls of ramen and udon, but for convenience, I preferred the cafeteria on campus that offered a different "set menu" meal each day that included a main dish with small sides. I was eating better food than I had most of my time in New York City. I wasn't overeating. I don't know how much weight I lost living in Japan, but it wasn't enough to need new clothes. After all, there were convenience and grocery stores and plenty of snacks.

When I returned to the United States, instead of going back to New York, I opted for a move to Los Angeles. I was hired to teach English as a Second Language at Los Angeles City College. The Los Angeles Community College District, a network of community colleges, required me to pass a physical examination before the semester began.

My new doctor, a well-muscled gay man catering mostly

to the gay community, took one look at my 38-inch waist and refused to sign off on my physical unless I lost at least 30 pounds. I'm almost six feet tall, and I carried it well but not well enough for my doctor and certainly not well enough for body-conscious Los Angeles. In my mind, I was very fat.

My doctor referred me to a nutritionist, an amazing woman who was the spitting image of the actress Meg Ryan. Together we studied an image of the food pyramid. According to her, the best eating plan ever. She put me on a reduced-calorie, low-fat, high-carbohydrate diet. Low-fat was all the rage at the time. I was limited to 1500 calories a day and could get them anywhere I liked. Since fat has double the calories of protein or carbohydrates per gram, fat was out, and carbs were in. After all, a calorie is a calorie, right? She showed me a 400-calorie portion of meat and a 400-calorie portion of beans. Which did I think would be more filling? The beans were a big pile, and the meat was pathetically small and dry. I opted for the beans. It worked. Most diets do work, and this one did.

Let's face it, lean meat is at best disappointing, at worst cardboard. About that time, a Hari Krishna guy on Venice Beach told me it took nine pounds of grain to make one pound of beef. I believed him. I considered what nine pounds of grain would look like—think of a single pound of ground meat—and the decision was obvious. As it was, I preferred the grain anyway. I decided to chuck meat altogether and become a vegetarian.

Along with my beans, salad, and veggies sprayed with fat-free artificial butter flavor, I ate a lot of rice, pasta, and bread—

all vegetarian. I faithfully had a large bowl of oatmeal every morning to bring down my cholesterol, which was already showing belligerence in my blood work. It never occurred to me that high LDL cholesterol was an odd thing to experience when I wasn't eating any meat or animal fat, which was the point of the heart-health hypothesis, misguided though it was. It didn't occur to my doctor either, who simply warned me off animal fat and didn't believe me when I told him I had opted to be vegetarian.

Now, of course, I understand that high cholesterol and triglycerides are a symptom of metabolic disease and, as you might well discover, not a product of consuming dietary fat. But of course, I thought I was eating a healthy diet, so the statin prescribed by my doctor was something I just accepted.

My only sources of real animal protein were egg whites (no yolks) and rubbery low-fat cheese. If you want to know what real disappointment is, think about having broccoli smothered in a cheesy sauce, then look at what happens when you cover broccoli with non-fat grated cheese!

I fully believe that eating the cheapest, most convenient foods triggered the weight gain that caused my Los Angeles doctor to look askance at my 38-inch waist. The low-calorie, low-fat, high-carbohydrate diet, given to me by my Meg Ryan lookalike, set me on the course for the diabetes diagnosis. I maintained the low-fat, high carbohydrate regimen as I had been advised by the nutritionist based on the food pyramid, which followed the recommendations of the Food and Drug Administration, causing my body to develop type 2 diabetes.

I originally lost weight on that diet, but after reaching my doctor's goal for my waistline, the weight crept back until, eventually, I weighed nearly 300 pounds, had a 48-inch waist, and was on two diabetes medications. I don't blame anyone, not even myself. All we did was follow the guidelines.

There was a personal shift in my eating habits when I went to college. I could easily blame myself for making the food choices I did. I could easily lay the blame on my budget, but honestly, even if I had more money, I don't know that I would have or even could have eaten better. Between shared kitchens and hungry fellow students, I probably did the best I could at the time.

There was also a societal shift during that time. The industry of food changed in the United States. Large industrial farms began buying out smaller farmers. Those farms where my parents bought eggs and meat don't really exist anymore. Processed foods began taking up more aisle space at supermarkets, and supermarkets doubled and tripled in size while neighborhood butchers and greengrocers became almost obsolete. It was just easier to get it all from the grocery store.

It's nearly impossible to avoid the connection between the establishment of the dietary guidelines in 1980, the Food and Drug Administration, and these significant changes. The power of industrial monoculture agriculture, farm bill subsidized commodity production, the interests of processed food manufacturers, and the rise of big pharma as an interest group form pieces of a jigsaw puzzle that fit nicely into a conspiracy theory puzzle.

I'm not so sure about the conspiracy part of it. I won't suggest intentional coordinated malfeasance, but there is enough circumstantial evidence of motive, means, and opportunity to warrant an indictment. I won't lay those charges. But I will say that these factors do fit together in a way that these interests found mutually profitable, unfortunately at the expense of the nation's health. Taking center stage are the dietary recommendations realized as the food pyramid, recommending a diet based not on meat and vegetables but grains, fruit, and vegetables. It is one that vilified meat and animal fat in favor of manufactured, chemically processed seed oils and an unsubstantiated notion that replaced culinary fat as a macronutrient with refined sugar and corn byproducts.

Evidence presented by Teicholz demonstrates that we took those recommendations to heart. In the end, instead of living healthier and longer, we ended up obese and riddled with type 2 diabetes.

I wonder what similarities you may have noticed between my experience and your own. What decisions did you make that were similar or different to mine? If you were born in the late fifties to early sixties, we probably have quite similar experiences, especially with dieting. You probably remember the debates over eggs being bad and then being good. If you were born in the late seventies, those dietary recommendations and the resulting glut of processed foods was the world you grew up in. In either case, let's now think about the epidemic levels of childhood obesity and type 2 diabetes. Let's do what we can to help our children and grandchildren develop and maintain a healthy, happy lifestyle.

Chapter 3:
Disease or Symptomatic Condition

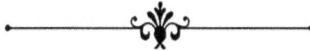

When I was a child, the only diabetic I knew was a type 1 diabetic. It was a fearful disease. In type 1 diabetes, the pancreas does not produce insulin. The life expectancy of someone with type 1 diabetes is dependent on early diagnosis, and, short of a successful pancreas transplant, their survival depends on their compliance with a treatment regimen that will last their entire lives.

Insulin, the hormone that regulates blood glucose, among other things, was discovered in 1921. And the first person to be treated with exogenous insulin was in 1922. Synthetic insulin was invented in 1978.

It is not hyperbole to say that the discovery of insulin and subsequent synthetic manufacture was nothing short of a miracle that took more than 50 years. It made diabetes a more manageable illness and prolonged the lives of many.

Type 2, or adult-onset diabetes, shares a similar faulty blood glucose regulation condition as type 1 but for a very different reason. In type 1 diabetes, the pancreas doesn't function. In type 2, the pancreas still functions, but the insulin produced is insufficient to keep blood glucose levels in check. There are two possible reasons for a pancreas not being up to the task. The first is seemingly the preferred option for allopathic medicine in that the pancreas is somehow damaged and needs help. Thus, medication is the response. The second is equally plausible: dietary choices generate too much glucose. Thus, dietary change is in order.

Indeed before diabetes medications and exogenous insulin injections, diabetes of all sorts was treated with dietary intervention. Even today, doctors suggest losing weight and increasing exercise *to help the medication!* In my mind, why not just help the pancreas? The thing I find disturbing is much of the information I am presenting has been around for decades. I ask myself, *If this science has been around for so long, why didn't my doctors tell me about it?* Much more disturbing a question might be if they didn't tell me, did they even know it? If they didn't know it, why not? If they did know it, well, that thought is the most disturbing.

My doctor did not have an answer for me when I asked how I had developed diabetes. He said I suffered from metabolic syndrome. When the allopathic medical community uses a word like syndrome, they intend to convey that they don't know the cause of the disease. A syndrome is a mystery defined by its symptoms or side effects.

Metabolic syndrome describes an array of conditions

that often occur comorbidly or simultaneously. Diabetes is one symptom. Obesity is another. Obesity, increased waist circumference, hypertension, elevated cholesterol and triglycerides, and an increased risk of cardiovascular risks for heart attack or stroke are all associated with metabolic syndrome. Gosh, have I not just named the biggest causes of death in Western society?

Traditionally, the obvious association between diabetes and obesity has been recognized. That is why my doctor suggested I lose weight, but he suggested I lose weight for just about everything. Any obese person knows exactly what I am talking about. Losing weight is a mantra the allopathic community constantly chants, including doctors who themselves are obese. If it's so easy to lose weight, Dr. Fatso, why aren't you doing it?

Many people, including many physicians, assume that obesity actually causes diabetes. That assumption, however, is wrong. Obesity and diabetes are often comorbid conditions. One may exacerbate the other. For example, if you inject insulin, you will likely gain weight. But to assume that one becomes diabetic because one is obese is not the case. A British comedian named Johnny Vegas once quipped on a panel show, *8 out of 10 Cats Does Countdown*, that he had been invited to speak at a diabetes society because they assumed he was diabetic because of his weight but he asserted, "I don't have it." Obesity does not cause type 2 diabetes. All obese people are not diabetic, and not all diabetics are fat.

The truth is very different. While obesity may precede a diagnosis of diabetes mellitus, it is not the cause. Obesity and diabetes are comorbid conditions of metabolic disease that can manifest in various conditions, including hypertension, heart disease, stroke, and a list of others. In my understanding, obesity and diabetes are *symptomatic conditions,* not the disease. Being overweight or obese is better understood as an often, but not always, early indicator of metabolic disease. But what if there were an even *earlier* sign of metabolic disease? What if the test for that symptom were as simple as routine blood work? And what if identification of that symptom exposed the underlying *cause* of metabolic syndrome? And, what if that cause were not some mysterious factors of genetics or luck but something in our environment? Finally, what if we could do something about it that didn't involve years of expensive pharmacological research?

Great news! That early symptom has been identified. There is still some room for genetic predisposition, but given the epidemic levels of metabolic disease, that predisposition, if one exists, is so prevalent in our species that it should be considered the norm and not the aberration. Upwards of at least 80% of the population is predisposed to developing metabolic disease. It is better said that the minority who do not suffer from metabolic disease is the exception to the rule.

This should be wonderful news to anyone walking around with a diagnosis of type 2 diabetes, prediabetes, metabolic disease, fatty liver, non-alcoholic cirrhosis of the liver, excess body fat, cardiovascular disease, and even hard to see visceral fat stored around organs behind the abdominal wall. It means we can actually do something to change the prognosis of metabolic disease. It does NOT have to be chronic or progressive.

The earliest symptomatic condition? Oh, didn't I say? Hyperinsulinemia. That is a big word for elevated insulin levels in the bloodstream. Fasting insulin measurements are as easy as a fasting glucose test, but elevated insulin levels can precede both increasing weight and high glucose levels by years, perhaps even decades. Why doctors do not routinely test for fasting insulin levels is a mystery. I can only guess, but my guess is a very cynical one. There's no real money in identifying hyperinsulinemia. There is no medication to control fasting insulin levels because if we control them medically, we would, in effect, be killing the patient. If we controlled insulin levels the way we controlled blood glucose levels, diabetics would rot from the inside out, like Lenny, only much faster. Pharmaceutical companies would rather treat high blood glucose levels, often by increasing insulin, which contributes to hyperinsulinemia. There's more money in it.

The truth is the treatment for hyperinsulinemia is absolutely free and requires no medical intervention beyond routine blood testing to see if it exists.

Some 17 years after my initial diagnosis of diabetes mellitus, I had been taking two medications—metformin and glimepiride—for several years. At my semi-annual check-up, my doctor revealed that my A1c was near 10, the highest it had ever been! He wanted me to begin taking a third medication before resorting to insulin injections. I give him credit for not pushing me into insulin injections at that point. I really do believe he had what he assumed was my best interests at heart.

I asked him to give me a list of medication possibilities as I wanted to read about my choices. As a clinical hypnotist,

I often look up the medications my clients take. I'm not a doctor. I don't prescribe medications but understanding how my clients' medications can affect them is essential in my work with them. I once had a client call in a frantic state about the uncontrollable emotions she was experiencing. She thought that hypnotherapy was making her crazy. Hypnosis can't make someone crazy, and though a session may be an emotional experience, the more common reaction is very positive.

I looked up her file and noticed she was taking synthetic thyroid medication. "Have you seen your doctor recently?" She said she had. "Did she change your thyroid medication in some way?" The dosage had been changed, and I suggested she call her doctor and explain what was happening.

I always ask about medications and the things for which my clients are being treated because it can truly play into what we do and how we work together. I'm mostly concerned about psychotropic medications for anxiety, depression, and attention disorders. These have little impact on our work, but a change in medications or dosages can cause dramatic emotional shifts. If I notice an antipsychotic medication that perhaps treats schizophrenia, the way I work with clients can be somewhat limited and requires a frank conversation with the client and maybe a release to speak with the prescribing physician.

"If you read about them, you won't want to take any of them," my doctor quipped as he gave me the list.

He was right. I didn't want to take any of them. I felt trapped. I blamed myself. Had I not been good enough?

Should I have exercised more? What was wrong with me? Was it really down to the simple carbohydrate pasta instead of that disgusting whole wheat pasta that tastes like sawdust? In those 17 years, I developed high blood pressure, took a statin, ate copious amounts of oatmeal for my cholesterol, and even acquired a skin condition that just appeared out of nowhere. I sunk into a hopeless depression for more than a month.

Like many other diabetics, I had long been barraged by online advertisements for prescription medications, miracle cures, superfoods, nutritional supplements, and a playlist of suggestions about diabetes. With the recent news from my doctor, I began watching some of the videos. I admit many of them were transparent in the promotion of those same superfoods, nutritional supplements, and miracle cures. Despite being able to recognize the manipulative sales lingo, I sank further. I wanted to believe them. I wanted to think that there was some food I could eat that would take care of me, that would clean the sugar out of my blood and let me keep my pasta. I hated myself for watching those videos and even clicking on the links to see how much the products cost, thus releasing a future flood of other links, advertisements, and spam emails.

I got lucky. One of my video feed suggestions was a documentary presentation on the trial of Dr. Tim Noakes. He was accused of unprofessional behavior because he had made a public statement recommending a low-carb and high-fat diet. I was captivated by his very logical and rational, science-based defense. I listened intently, and I can admit now that the high-fat part of the diet scared me. It made me doubt and question his reasoning. It went against virtually everything I thought I knew about diet and nutrition. Yet, I was captivated. He backed up everything he said with sound, reliable science. His demeanor was so matter of fact, seemingly so confident, that I was impressed by his composure. A book about his trial, *Real Food on Trial*, is listed in the suggested reading and is well worth the read.

What I got out of that video was that there was something else, something other than what I had heard from my doctor and the nutritionist about how to live with diabetes. It was so vastly different that I knew I needed to investigate more. I wasn't ready to simply jump in because some physician from South Africa got into trouble promoting it, but I could look into it with an open but cautious mind.

I then stumbled on a book by Dr. Ken Berry, *Lies My Doctor Told Me*. I admit the title got my attention. I never thought my doctor had lied to me, but it was quite possible he either didn't know or didn't believe the things I was reading about. In his book, Berry exposes many of the myths commonly held by those in the health industry. Many of those myths were directly or indirectly related to my condition. Berry, too, cites real science but explains it in terms accessible to most people. He also takes time to exhort physicians in practice to investigate the science behind the assumptions they might be making.

I later discovered Berry had a YouTube channel, and impressively he commonly tells his viewers not to simply take his word for it but to look at the science he cites. Here was confirmation that there was another way of seeing things and that the recommendations and advice I had been given were not the only ones out there. My hope and resolve were strengthened.

The idea of taking my health into my own hands was both exciting and scary at the same time. Could I believe my doctor or not? Could I trust the advice of my physician? The ultimate answer was an emphatic yes and no. My doctor knew far more than I did, and even if his information was a bit out of date, it was better than something I might get by googling questions. At the same time, I became painfully aware that I needed to make informed decisions about my doctor's advice. Those informed decisions needed to be based on science, not merely assumptions.

All my searching and querying brought another YouTube video into my feed. It was a recording of a presentation made by Dr. Jason Fung at a medical conference. There he stood, lecturing a room full of physicians on therapeutic intermittent fasting. One of the things he said made me laugh. He said we never see a reunion show of The Biggest Loser. He is right. Most of those contestants have regained the weight they lost. He blamed this fact on *how* they lost weight, a dramatically reduced-calorie diet, and extreme exercise.

He went on to illustrate insulin resistance by talking about how in the Tokyo subways, attendants literally shove passengers into trains because they are overcrowded. I was there. I had been shoved! I got what he was saying about insulin and how the doctor treated my diabetes, like those Japanese subway attendants shoving glucose into my overstuffed cells. It all made sense! He quoted study after scientific study, impressing me the way Noakes and Berry had.

Here were real scientists and physicians who were openly calling into question the advice my physician and the nutritionist had given me. I felt like a bird that had been stunned from flying into a window. I was caught completely off guard.

I wondered if the advice to cut carbohydrates and fast hadn't been proffered simply because people wouldn't listen to it. After all, nobody wants to fast, and nobody wants to cut carbs. On the other hand, shouldn't I have been told about these strategies, at least, by the nutritionist, even if only as an option? Did they think I could not or would not follow that advice? Or was it that they didn't know about that advice? Or were they blinded from that advice because of their training or belief?

I once had a client say that she felt lucky finding me because when she asked her neurologist about consulting a hypnotist, the neurologist said she didn't believe in hypnosis because it was against her religion. What kind of criteria apart from science do some doctors use for offering treatment options?

I had the sense I was embarking on a dangerous journey. I was going to go rogue. I was going to try fasting and reducing my carbohydrates. I had the feeling that if I told my doctor what I was doing, he might not approve or he might try to talk me out of it, or he might insist on that third medication. So, I did not tell him. I just never got back to him about that third medication. I had another appointment with him scheduled four months later. I'd decide what to tell him then.

I now believe that many of the conditions treated directly by our medical system are really symptomatic conditions of metabolic disease and not diseases in their own right springing out of genetic predispositions or unknowable sources. I admit that many of these conditions are serious enough to earn the distinction of a disease, but it is easier for me to wrap my mind around my own wellness plan to see them as symptomatic conditions that may well be temporary if we can turn things around.

Many of the most dangerous, life-threatening conditions, indeed many of the biggest causes of death in our society, stem directly from the shift in our culture that was brought about by those dietary recommendations that instructed us to base our dietary habits on cheap, subsidized, processed carbohydrates.

But like Dr. Ken Berry instructs, I don't want you to believe me. I am not a doctor, and I cannot offer medical advice to anyone under any circumstances. I hope you decide to read, learn, research, and make informed decisions with which you are comfortable. If you prefer to keep it simple and blindly accept the advice of your physician, great. Do that. I honestly hope you have a good one, not merely a well-intentioned one.

Chapter 4:
The Initial Plan

⸻⫯⸻

I have to call this chapter the initial plan because my plan to address my diabetes evolved. In the beginning, I knew very little. I had heard a lot, read some things, had hope in what I had learned but would it pan out *for me*? Even more to the point, what *exactly* should I do?

Sustainability is a buzzword, and from the outset, I had the idea that any changes I would make had to be sustainable. At the time, to me, that meant permanent. I thought whatever I did, I had to maintain it forever. Come to think of it, it was a reasonable assumption. Diets had worked for me, but the results were temporary. I didn't understand why this was happening beyond blaming myself for returning to my old ways. That's not an unfair assumption, but the self-recrimination part is vile.

The diet and exercise industry cultivates the idea that if a diet or exercise plan doesn't work or doesn't work permanently, it's the fault of the dieter. Fad diet after fad diet promises amazing results, but the diet industry would disappear if those plans worked permanently. Consider all the supplements, magic pills, superfoods, and exercise equipment sold to the American public. If they work at all, the effect isn't permanent. But the patrons of this industry have been trained to blame themselves for not maintaining their gains.

Some hypnotists, members of my own industry, also take advantage of this phenomenon. People lose weight with hypnotists and then go off on their own and gain it back. Most don't blame the hypnotist; they blame themselves, and so they come back. I suppose, in most ways, this is normal. If everyone who ever bought a gym membership actually used it consistently, the gym would go out of business. I know people who have gone to Weight Watchers, Nutrisystem, and Medical Weight Loss clinics more than once. My personal ethics don't allow for such strategies. I prefer to build sustainability into my work as best I can.

For years, I came under criticism from some of my peers because my smoking cessation program is four sessions long rather than a single session. I was trained to help people quit smoking in a single session and did that successfully for perhaps the first year of my practice.

But then I discovered that some of my clients had gone back to smoking weeks or months later and, perhaps reasonably, had blamed themselves. I wondered how many clients of mine had done just that and how many of my peers' clients were also doing similar.

My integrity meter told me I should be able to do more for them to increase the likelihood of sustainable success. Of course, I could not control what people did after our work was done, but there had to be something more I could do for them. In response, I created my four-session program. I charge about the same rate as other well-skilled hypnotists do for a single smoking cessation session. I am happy to say that the success rate is a sustainable 95%. It's not 100%, and that's why I can't make guarantees. My integrity no longer allows me to offer single session "miracles." My plan is sustainable, and I back it up with a promise, not a guarantee. I offer my clients a lifetime promise. If at any time they feel really tempted to smoke another cigarette for any reason, I ask them to promise to speak with me first. This option is open to them for the rest of my life, no matter how long it's been since we worked together.

So, as I began my journey, I knew *or thought I knew* that whatever changes I would make if they worked, would have to be permanent. I later learned that once substantial gains are made, people gain some wiggle room, but by the time they get that wiggle room, they don't often really want to wiggle as much as they thought they would.

My primary concern was diabetes and getting my blood glucose levels under control. I decided that I would experiment on myself. I did not know the term **biohacking** at the time, but that was what I had planned. I would test my blood glucose regularly, hoping to notice trends. I was initially interested in several readings. I planned testing when I woke up, at noon, just before dinner, and before going to bed. I later tested more aggressively, but that came later.

I knew that I had to cut my carbohydrate consumption, so I started by cutting them in half. Whatever I would typically eat, I would eat only half. Being a card-carrying member of the clean plate club, I struggled emotionally with how to do this. My father frequently encouraged us to take all we wanted during our meals but eat all we had taken. At first, I struggled to leave food on the plate. A little later, I'd serve myself a plate and put half the carbohydrates back before beginning to eat. Then I figured out how much to take in the first place.

About two weeks in, I found myself cutting carbs a bit more. Instead of being wrapped in bread, I could enjoy a sandwich with a knife and a fork. It wasn't worth cooking half an ear of corn for myself when I could eat a salad instead. The part of the baked potato I really enjoyed was the skin, so I waited until my husband had polished off the potato and offered me the skin. One day we ordered pizza, and I found myself scraping the topping off the crust and was more than satisfied just eating the toppings. And yes, someone else reached for my crusts.

I am not going to pretend this process was easy. I went through a lot of mental reevaluating. I first looked for healthier substitutes for the carbohydrates I was eating. Because many people on YouTube make keto cooking videos, I bought ingredients that were astronomically expensive. I made bread in mugs in my microwave, following recipes that required six eggs for a loaf of bread. I tried to make noodles from alternative flours, eggs, and even gelatin. I didn't go completely crazy with keto ingredients but bought xanthan gum mostly because the quantities needed were so minute. I instinctively disliked the overly processed ingredients like whey protein isolates and other things I would not typically want to consume. Eventually, I gave up in frustration. The emerging keto products in the markets were so highly processed that I avoided them instinctively, especially after reading the list of ingredients. I tried to stay close to real food as much as possible.

Despite all I heard about calories not being important, I still had that calorie model in my head. I was still afraid of the calories in fat, so in replacing the bulk on my plate chose to fill it with non-starchy vegetables. The simplest way of identifying good veggies, I discovered, was any vegetable that grew above ground was less likely to be starchy or higher in carbohydrates. The big exception, of course, is corn. It hurt a bit when I realized corn was a grain, not a vegetable, and had to be considered a carbohydrate. Aarrgh! Sadly, the same went for fruit.

I chose to read about and try to understand the medications I was taking. The first was metformin. When I looked it up, it seemed harmless. The article I read said that it increased insulin sensitivity but didn't say how. It also inhibits sugar absorption in the intestines. Exactly what did that mean? Was I just going to pee or poo the sugar out? And thirdly, it would inhibit my body from creating glucose and releasing it into the bloodstream.

My second medication was glimepiride. This drug, a sulfonylurea, supports and increases the body's own insulin production. Because of the increase in insulin production, the drug comes with a warning about low blood sugar. Given how high my blood sugar was, I did not think that was of much concern. (I later found out how wrong that assumption was.)

Never for a moment at this stage did I consider changing anything about my medications. I was avoiding going on a third medication. If anything, the medications I was already on weren't doing enough for me, so I'd keep them as is. Though I had heard testimonials about people who had stopped taking diabetes medications entirely, I did not for even a second hope for such a thing for myself. I really just wanted to get my diabetes under control.

In my college days, I attempted to fast for religious reasons. Back then, I hoped to be inspired in my spiritual journey. Fasting, in my mind, was self-denial, a sacrifice of something normal—eating. I thought of it as subduing my body, my carnal nature in preference to my spiritual being. All I really got was hungry. I was not at all excited about fasting.

I decided to see how long I fasted naturally. That is how long I naturally went without eating between my last bit of food one day and my first bit of food the next day. I quickly realized that I never went more than nine or 10 hours without eating something.

One day, while watching a video blog episode of a homesteading family, something sunk in. The husband of the family was walking his viewers through his daily chores. The video started early in the morning before dawn. He was feeding animals, checking on things around the farm, and working on a building project when he smiled into the camera and said it was time for breakfast.

He did all those things *before* breakfast! Wow! I let that sink in and began to think through what I might be able to accomplish before breakfast. Gradually my natural fasting time increased to between 14 and 16 hours.

I joined fasting and low-carb Facebook groups. Because those groups, while monitored, are generally populated by peers, some of the advice offered is pretty bad. One has to think through following advice from people in Facebook groups.

I subscribed to *Low-Carb Down Under* and *Low-carb USA* YouTube channels and quickly found myself getting more information from credible sources than I thought possible. The amount of information available immediately showed me how much I didn't know and how much I needed to learn. It was like becoming a student all over again.

I bought books and books. Thank heavens for audio versions. There aren't enough hours in a day to read all the books I bought and live a normal life at the same time. At least with audio, I could listen while I did other things. I've listed some of those books in the suggested reading section at the end of this book. I haven't listed everything I read for two reasons: Some of it was just dumb, unclear, or outright wrong. A lot of it was just repetitive. It took me quite a while to become a more selective consumer of that material.

Chapter 5:
The Best-Laid Plans

I had been testing my blood four times a day. When I woke up, my glucose levels were consistently above 110, the cutoff described to me by my doctor. They tended to drop during the day, but that mainly depended on when I ate. If the noon reading happened before lunch, my glucose levels would be lower but still above 100. If I tested after I ate something, I considered myself lucky if the readings were below 140.

Because I was trying to increase my natural fasting time, I was eating earlier and not snacking after dinner. One night after an exhausting day of work, back-to-back clients, no break, I put myself to bed without my dinner. I did not really feel hungry. I was just tired.

I woke up shortly after going to sleep, and I felt creepy,

really sick. I decided to test my blood, and the reading was the lowest one I had ever gotten, 62. I am glad I woke up! If I hadn't, my journey might well have been over.

We had some candied pineapple in the house. It wasn't my favorite thing to eat, which is why I had left it alone, but it was the quickest access to sugar available. I ate two pieces and almost instantly felt better.

Despite being tired, I lay awake, almost afraid to sleep again. It was confirmation that in doing what I was doing, I was taking my life into my own, mostly ignorant, inexperienced hands. At the same time, I thought that I needed to do just that. I can't say it enough. What my doctor and the nutritionist did for me helped, but it was not enough. Not for me.

I imagined the low blood glucose level was because I had not eaten since early that day combined with the sulfonylurea, which increased insulin and carried a warning about low blood sugar. It was a reasonable assumption, but if I continued doing what I was doing, wouldn't my medication have to change? Dare I ask my doctor to help me with this?

I didn't want to talk to him. I didn't think he would approve of my experiment. I knew he wouldn't want to be even tangentially responsible for it. I was on my own. Granted, the day had been unusually busy, and I hadn't eaten but shouldn't my body be able to handle that? I came up with two criteria for continuing my journey.

I didn't think I was getting enough information from my testing schedule, and I needed to test my blood glucose readings in a more methodical and informative fashion. I decided to test my blood more often. In addition to testing in the morning, I'd test again just before my first bite of the day, thinking the latter was a more representative number of my true fasting glucose levels.

I had noticed that my blood sugar levels very often went up for that first reading of the day. That seemed illogical since I had not eaten anything at all for more than 12 hours. I asked about this curious factor in a Facebook group, and someone suggested I look up the *dawn phenomenon*.

Apparently, in preparation for morning activities, the liver engages in gluconeogenesis; that is, it makes and releases glucose into the bloodstream. Good news on that end, but the abnormally high levels of those readings also indicated that insulin resistance was at play. For me, that morning reading became a gauge of insulin resistance, not really fasting glucose.

I would also test at 30, 60, and 120 minutes after eating. This process did two things for me. First, it prohibited me from grazing after a meal. I had to wait at least two hours before putting anything in my mouth. More importantly, when combined with a memory of what I had eaten and how much, this series of readings became an indicator of how I reacted to certain foods and showed me when my postprandial (after eating) blood glucose would reach its apex.

I continued to test my blood glucose before going to bed. I often used every finger on both hands once a day. Sometimes I missed readings, but in general, I did pretty well. I saved the spreadsheet as evidence for my doctor when I would see him next.

The sulfonylurea warned about low blood sugar, so I would cut it in half and see what happened, but I would leave the metformin dosage intact.

Surprisingly, there wasn't much of a jump in readings even after a few days of cutting that pill in half. I expected them to go up significantly, but they were only slightly higher and quickly dropped to the previous levels. I took that as a very positive sign.

I continued cutting carbs mostly because I wasn't craving them anymore. It almost became silly to prepare them. The wheat four, rice, oatmeal, in fact, all grains nearly completely disappeared from my pantry.

I don't know if I lost weight in the first month. I wasn't concerned about my weight and didn't weigh myself. Actually, I didn't weigh myself for several months until a colleague across the hall pulled me aside.

"You are really losing weight," he said.

"I suppose so."

"No supposing about it. Congratulations, but you need to go shopping. You're a professional, and this,"—gesturing to my outfit—"just looks sloppy."

He was right. At the time he spoke to me, I had lost some eight inches off my waist. I had already drilled several new holes in my belt. I was putting off shopping because I wasn't yet done. I did go shopping, and honestly, it was fun. For the first time in years and years, I was able to buy clothes in a regular store that didn't cater to large men. That was marvelous.

Chapter 6:
How Sweet It Isn't

————— ❧ —————

In 2014 I went a whole year without added sugar. I had watched the documentary *Fed Up*, narrated by Katie Couric, which exposed the exponential infiltration of sugar into the American diet. The video featured pediatric endocrinologist Robert Lustig who described sugar as an addictive "dose-dependent hepatotoxin." Those are big words for liver poison. A little poison might be okay, but the more you consume, the greater the toxicity.

Today, sugar addiction is bantered about almost flippantly. Some people actually seem proud of it, happily scarfing chocolate bars, ice cream cones, and donuts. In my practice, I get calls about it several times a month. The addiction is real, and while hypnosis can help a person manage the cravings and control the urges, it can't simply undo a chemical addiction.

But, sugar addiction carries a *double* whammy. Consuming sugar creates nearly the same response in the brains as does cocaine, but it's more insidious—it's programmed into our physiology.

Back in the days when sweet things were available only when fruit and berries happened to be ripe in our climate when discovered, those foods triggered indulgent behavior. The rare treat of something sweet naturally helped our bodies store a little fat for leaner times. And let's be honest here. Outside of extreme poverty, truly lean times such as famine are rare in today's world. Even in extreme poverty, the availability of fast, easy junk food is cheap enough, and virtually all of it is laced with addicting sugar additives.

In quantities other than scant, the liver toxicity of consuming sugar is a matter of science. Millions of people with type 2 diabetes stand as testimony, but many more suffer from fatty liver disease and non-alcoholic cirrhosis of the liver, obesity, hyperinsulinemia, high blood pressure, and cardiovascular disease, all of which are directly related to metabolic disease.

According to the New Hampshire Department of Health and Human Services, the average American consumes 152 pounds of sugar a year. That is more than twelve and a half pounds in a single month! Compare that to 200 years ago, when it was estimated that an average American might consume two pounds of sugar in an entire *year!*

According to my mother, who was born in 1920, a piece of fruit was a rare treat when she was young. A single orange was something children got in their Christmas stocking, along with some nuts in the shell and maybe a few pieces of hard candy. By the 1960s, my Halloween haul was a substantial pile of candy. But even then, when we consumed sugar, we knew it. It was candy or cake, and it was still a rare treat.

Today, the problem isn't just that we eat too much candy, how much sugar we put in our morning coffee, or even how much sugar is in a can of soda pop. Sugar, in various chemical forms derived from beets, corn, and cane sugar, has found its way into just about every processed or manufactured food in the United States. There are some fifty different names for those sugar derivatives that enhance flavor and surreptitiously nurture and play on sugar addiction, getting us to use more, eat more and, of course, buy more.

That documentary angered and inspired me. I stopped using sugar in my home. I forbade myself candy, cookies, cakes, and desserts. I purged my pantry of processed and packaged foods that contained added sugars of any kind. That was rough and expensive, but I was determined to fight back against the barrage of sugar in my diet.

Almost immediately, the cravings flared out of control. Talk about withdrawal! I wasn't yet a practicing hypnotist back then, and the only way I knew to address a craving was to satisfy it in the healthiest possible way or tough it out cold turkey. In the first several weeks of my no-added-sugar project, I ate copious amounts of fresh fruit. Fruit juice was out because of its concentration. A glass of orange juice might be equivalent to five or six oranges! I'd rather have the orange anyway. I didn't think or realize how concentrated the sugars were in dried fruit like raisins and never thought about how some processors might actually coat dried fruit in sugar. The box of raisins didn't last long, but I didn't buy another one.

Eventually, the cravings eased a bit, but I think that happened mostly because there were times when I had simply run out of fruit and had to muscle my way through the cravings. They eased, but they never stopped—for a whole year! I hadn't cut my carbs because, thanks to that nutritionist, I didn't see complex carbohydrates in the same category as sugar. I probably ate a lot more carbohydrates but figured my main battle was against sugar. After all, as long as they were complex carbohydrates and composed less than 60% of my calories, I was in the safe zone, right? Whole wheat bread slathered in margarine sprinkled with cinnamon and an artificial sweetener made perfect sense to me back then.

The feelings of self-imposed deprivation and denial never left. As I look back on my experience, I treated it like a diet. I lost 40 pounds that year but began gaining it back the moment I reached my one-year goal, loosening up on the food choices. My slippery slope was made of sugar. Those hard-won 40 pounds returned with a vengeance, and I tacked on another 20 pounds for good measure.

One of the things I did not understand back in 2014 was the difference between fructose and sucrose. This is important in addressing metabolic disease. Sugar contains two sweet parts: fructose and sucrose. Sucrose, like all carbohydrates, is converted immediately into glucose by the body. The consumption of sucrose and carbohydrates immediately raises blood glucose levels. While fructose does not affect blood sugar levels like sucrose and carbohydrates do, it must be processed by the liver, which means to me that when we consume fructose, whether directly in fruit or processed in the form of high fructose corn syrup, we are unnecessarily taxing the liver.

Of course, in 2014, I hadn't targeted elevated insulin as a problem. I wasn't even focused on blood glucose levels. After all, my diabetes medication was doing a fair enough job of controlling blood sugar at the time.

I had been drinking diet soda pop for years, believing that I was saving calories and avoiding sugar. But there was a catch of which I was blissfully unaware. I didn't understand something called the *cephalic insulin response*. The tongue tastes sweetness and sends a signal to the brain that something sweet is being consumed. The brain relays the message to the stomach, the liver, and the pancreas to expect sugar. The stomach gets the juices going. The liver stops gluconeogenesis and gets ready for the job of processing yet more excess glucose. And the pancreas starts kicking out insulin. When useless, unrecognizable chemicals arrive in the stomach without the promised sugar, the stomach, liver, and pancreas send an urgent message to the brain asking what happened to the sugar they were expecting. While the mind knows about artificial, non-nutritive sweeteners, the brain only recognizes that something has gone wrong. It automatically begins triggering cravings for food that will supply the sugar to cope with the excess insulin. Perhaps another slice of that whole wheat bread, a bag of chips, or even a fat-free cookie that, despite its promises of health, is nothing but cheap, processed carbohydrates and chemicals

Not only was I consuming non-nutritive sweet-tasting chemicals that have proven health risks and which the body does not recognize as food, but I was triggering insulin when it was not needed contributing to hyperinsulinemia and thus possibly worsening my metabolic disease by further cultivating insulin resistance.

These days, sugar of any kind has minimal use in our home. I admit it exists, as does a jar of dehydrated stevia leaves from a plant I nurtured for a year or so. The sugar is used rarely. I make kombucha, which is fermented tea. The fermentation process consumes most if not all of the sugar. The beverage doesn't taste sweet like the commercial varieties, which are loaded with added sugar. We may drink kombucha several times a month as a special beverage with a meal. At that rate, that dose-dependent hepatotoxin doesn't get very far in our lives.

I have used the stevia leaves so rarely that I don't know why I bother keeping them, except I nurtured that plant through two winters to get that harvest and dehydrated the leaves myself. It's more sentimental than anything. I never use them.

One thing I've noticed is that my taste for sweet things has definitely changed. I generally won't indulge in desserts beyond a single bite. At that, I usually taste something just to be polite when we've been invited to dinner, and I wish to legitimize my praise of the entire meal. My hosts don't seem to mind if I don't eat dessert, and they appreciate my telling them that it was delicious. It's only a little fib. It was likely too sweet for my taste, and I base my compliment mostly on the praises of everyone else at the table.

I have the wiggle to eat a dessert now and again but don't really want to use it. When I take a bite or two, usually off my husband's plate, just about everything I taste is cloyingly sweet, too sweet to actually enjoy. I'm much happier with a few fresh berries in full-fat Greek yogurt or unsweetened whipped cream. In the summer, we drink a lot of hibiscus mint tea. Hibiscus is naturally tart, so I imagine the sweetness comes from the mint, but neither of these herbs has sugar. I once put a stevia leaf into that tea, and it was too sweet for me to enjoy it, though my husband loved it.

Just the other day, we were having dinner with friends, and there was a wonderful, beautiful raspberry cheesecake. There we were, all in the kitchen, trying out a new whipped cream dispenser with a charger, like an old-fashioned seltzer bottle. The recipe called for two cups of heavy cream, some vanilla, and *six tablespoons of powdered sugar*. They only put in half of the sugar, but it was still too sweet for me. I would have preferred it with just the cream and the vanilla. I tasted a bit off my husband's plate. (He doesn't really mind.) The cheesecake and the whipped cream were quite good but too sweet for me.

These days, I rarely have any craving for sweet things. I'm not immune to the *memory* of those cravings, but I'm almost always disappointed with the actual taste when I give in. A more recent adaptation to my psychological strategy for avoiding sweets is the threat of loss of the enjoyment of the memory.

On a recent trip to visit friends in New Jersey, we entered

a family diner to have lunch. At the cashier's stand, there was a display case of enticingly beautiful cakes, pies, and other confections. I felt a kind of exhilaration at seeing that display. For a few moments, I felt like a child again.

I knew that everyone in our group would be partaking in some sort of dessert; after all, we were celebrating. We hadn't seen one another for the two years we had been in Covid-19 isolation. I could order one with them, and we might all share, but I would eat only a bite of each, including my own. What a schemer I was at that moment!

Enjoying the good company and our meal together, a thought occurred to me, *You know you will be disappointed when you try those desserts.* I knew it was true. My tastes had actually changed, and I was thoroughly familiar with that disappointment. Thinking of the enjoyment I felt when I first saw that display case, I realized that I would lose that feeling forever once I tasted the delicacies on offer. I decided to forego tasting any of them on the prospect of guarding that childlike joy I experienced. That joy was worth more to me than any bite of a dessert. From that point forward, I chose to see such things on offer, cherishing the youth harbored in my heart. I realized I didn't need to eat any of it.

Chapter 7:
Thank You, Keto People

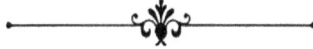

———•◦❦◦•———

O ne does not get very deep into the low-carb movement without being surrounded by people extolling the ketogenic diet. Indeed, low-carb and keto are almost the same thing. People following a ketogenic diet generally restrict their carbohydrate consumption to a specific percentage of their diet or a specific number of grams of carbohydrates per day. In my past dieting life, I've counted calories, units, points, portions, and servings. I hate diet counting! The very thought of calculating the macros found in a serving of food or a recipe is mind-numbingly tedious to me. I can do it. I have done it occasionally, but I hate it.

In the years I've been deleting my diabetes, I've learned a lot of recipes and created a good many of my own. Of course, I've shared them with my clients when it seemed right to do so.

More than a few have suggested creating a website, vlog, or even a cookbook. The reason I do not take on the task is simple. I don't want to calculate macros per serving. That would almost take the fun out of eating anything for me.

Although I am in and out of ketosis all the time, I do not follow a strict ketogenic diet. I don't test for ketosis often. Neither do I much consider the depth of ketosis when I do. I'm either in or out. That's enough for me. I have the strips in my bathroom, and more often than not, they expire before I use them all. Ketosis meters, which look like blood glucose monitors, are expensive, and the test strips for those are obscenely too expensive for most people to afford. After all, the knowledge gained seems minimal to me.

The main advantage of knowing one is in ketosis is simple; we know that our body is using fat as fuel. Remember, the body stores energy in two forms. Glycogen is stored in the liver, and when glycogen stores are full, the liver converts excess glucose into fat. When we combine a reduced carbohydrate diet with intermittent therapeutic fasting, our body first uses the glucose in our cells. Activity levels contribute to how quickly this happens, but I'll treat that topic in greater detail later. Then the liver starts converting glycogen into glucose. That is called gluconeogenesis. Once glycogen stores are depleted, the body begins to access fat for energy. If this happens with any degree of regularity, the body's default is to begin creating ketones instead of glucose.

Nutritional ketosis is the state we reach when our diet strictly restricts carbohydrates, and our protein intake is moderate. In the absence of sufficient glucose, the need for insulin drops, and the liver begins producing ketones. Your body functions as well on ketones as it does glucose. Some say it functions even better. In my experience, I have less hunger, fewer cravings, more energy, and a clearer mind when I'm in moderate ketosis.

I don't know why people are afraid of ketosis. On one of my visits to my doctor, he asked for a urine sample, something we hadn't tested at the lab. Apart from being charged for the test, which I considered unfair since it would have been included with my lab work, I gladly peed in the cup. I saw him later that week by accident, and we spoke casually.

"We got the results back from that urine sample. There were ketones in it."

I brightened. "Great, that's good news." His reaction was difficult to read. He seemed astonished or at least puzzled by my comfort with ketones. I didn't understand his reaction at all. So, I did some research, which is pretty much my default mode when it comes to metabolic health. I have only found a few easily debunked arguments against prolonged deep ketosis and only one against ramping it up.

Some people experience a kind of *keto flu* when the liver begins ramping up ketosis or, better said, when it switches from normally making glucose to primarily making ketones. I experienced it without realizing it one day when I felt like I was coming down with a cold. I was a little tired, a little achy, and just felt like doing nothing. I trudged through my day.

I had been curious about ketosis and purchased the test strips, which are inexpensive plastic strips with a tiny bit of absorbent material at one end. You put the material end into your urine stream, and if it changes color, you are producing measurable ketones. The darker it gets, the more ketones that are present. At the time, I was testing for ketones after every fast, including my regular natural fast. My feelings of coming down with a cold happened between two tests, and the second one indicated the presence of ketones.

If you bring up the ketogenic diet among naysayers, someone will usually mention *ketoacidosis*. Ketoacidosis is a serious condition but is primarily a danger for type 1 diabetics. Ketoacidosis happens in the *absence* of insulin, and in type 1 diabetics, insulin can be an issue because the pancreas does not function properly. If your pancreas creates insulin and you eat vegetables, which naturally contain small amounts of carbohydrate, and if you eat meat, a portion of which is converted to glucose anyway, you likely need not worry about ketoacidosis.

There seems to be some correlation between kidney disease and eating a high-protein diet, as some ketogenic diet folks do. I'm no expert on kidney disease or even the ketogenic diet, but I do know that a ketogenic diet does not necessarily mandate a high protein diet. The direction is to reduce carbs, not eat all the protein they can shove into their mouths. In the low-carb and high-fat model, caloric deficit may be more than made up by using healthy fat, not necessarily extra protein. If one is looking to add bulk, it might be better to look toward organic above-ground vegetables because vegetables that grow below ground are often starchier than those that grow above.

In the research science community, there seems to be some

conflation between a very high protein diet and nutritional ketosis. I suspect it comes from people's almost automatic association between the Atkins diet and the ketogenic diet. While I don't know enough about the Atkins diet to form an opinion on it perse, I take umbrance with thinking a ketogenic diet involves copious increases in protein. The sheer number of people in deep nutritional ketosis who eat a moderate protein diet seem to have no trouble.

I'll just point out here that it sometimes helps to learn who paid for the study when reading scientific studies. Knowing the funding sources can be quite revealing about the way the results of the study are presented. Often studies are funded surreptitiously through a gift or endowment to a university or through the underwriting of the journal that published the results.

Finally, the most credible of the arguments is that remaining in deep nutritional ketosis over a long period of time may cause your body to grow accustomed to *not* using much insulin. Those in very deep ketosis for a long time may temporarily experience high blood glucose levels after consuming carbohydrates in quantities that have become abnormal for them. Even in these unusual circumstances, the impact seems to be temporary. I doubt the body would completely forget how to direct blood glucose, but I imagine it is possible for it to become sluggish. Eventually, the body remembers insulin, and while they might be knocked out of ketosis, the problem doesn't last, and they can go back into ketosis quite easily.

I'll also include one more caution that I learned through

a client. In the low-carb and high-fat diet, some people consume so much fat that the fat they are eating becomes the primary source of fat for conversion into ketones. By this, I mean the person is eating so much fat that the liver has no reason to access body fat to produce ketones. It's the ketogenic version of treading water, staying afloat but not getting anywhere. Forgive me for being a bit graphic here but if you notice an oily surface on the water in your toilet before flushing after a poo, cut back on the fat.

We can hasten ketone production with fasting and increased activity. In my routine, light ketosis is common. It depends, of course, on what and how much I have eaten. I don't track it constantly as many ketogenic followers do. I am certain to be in ketosis if I do a 24-hour fast because my regular diet is rather low in carbohydrates. If I choose to do an even longer fast, I'm increasing ketosis throughout that fast. If I break a longer fast with a moderate protein and higher fat meal that avoids carbohydrates, I remain in ketosis even longer, sometimes for a day or more after the fast.

Celebrity trainer Jillian Michaels from the television show *The Biggest Loser* has made public statements against the ketogenic diet, suggesting it is not a healthy diet. I wonder what evidence she had to make such a claim because I can't find any that wasn't clearly biased in favor of processed or manufactured foods or that the processed food industry funded.

I will admit that when I heard her say that I had already come to believe that her method, the one she used in *The Biggest Loser*, that of strict calorie restriction and punishing physical activity, was *extremely unhealthy*, especially in the long run. Since the show is no longer on the air, I wonder who is sponsoring her professional career now. Perhaps I'm being unfairly snide and overly skeptical, but in practicality, the only thing unhealthy about a ketogenic diet is the crazy ways in which some people apply the principles in their own ignorance. That is, without understanding what they are doing and how it affects their bodies.

As for me, I owe the ketogenic community a great deal of gratitude. The plethora of YouTube channels focused on ketogenic recipes helped me reduce carbohydrates at the beginning of my journey. At the time, living without bread or pasta was inconceivable to me. If abandoning carbohydrates completely were a criterion for beginning my journey, I think I would not have even taken the first step. I wasn't ready for that change, and much less did I ever think it possible.

Of course, I initially craved bread, pasta, and especially crunchy snacks. Ketogenic cooks showed me ways of having those things with fewer carbs. I'll reveal that many of the replacement recipes were disappointing, and I tried recipe after recipe in desperation of finding something that really worked for me. Gradually, I came to terms with not really needing bread, pasta, or rice.

While I am a pretty decent cook, I struggled to create things that had a real crunch without breading, grains, and deep-frying. I found cheese cracker recipes online and tried substituting garbanzo bean flour for wheat flour, saving me significant carbohydrates. It worked because gluten wasn't important in the recipe, but those carbohydrates added up. Through the ketogenic community, I learned about making flaxseed crackers and cheese crisps that needed no flour whatsoever.

Recipes for chaffles and ninety-second microwave mug bread helped me get over the loss of bread in my life. I still enjoy chaffles, though mug bread has gone by the wayside.

The downside to many ketogenic recipes is that they often require odd, uncommon, expensive, and highly processed ingredients. For me, it has to be real food for it to be even considered food.

It seems to me that many adherents to the ketogenic diet don't actually want to change; they just want to lose weight. Obesity is only one symptomatic condition of metabolic disease. Merely addressing the symptom and not the cause is little more than a bandaid. What about all the other symptomatic conditions? In my opinion, addressing the root cause of metabolic disease is of the utmost importance, and processed food is part of the problem, even if that processed food has the right macros.

The market has been flooded with what I call *keto krap*. A product labeled "keto-friendly" doesn't mean it is healthy. Of course, in our supermarkets, *any* product that proclaims its own health value is likely to be misleading. Keto cookies, keto candy, keto chips, keto crackers, keto bread, keto ice cream, and keto desserts are too often packed with chemically modified ingredients, artificial flavors, artificial sweeteners, cheap oils, emulsifiers, and bulk ingredients that ostensibly add fiber, thus supposedly cutting down the carbs. Food manufacturers have taken a good thing, the ketogenic diet, and turned it into a fad-diet marketing strategy. Shame on them. Of course, what can you expect from an industry with seemingly no shame at all? Oh, I'm not talking about everyone involved in the industry but the industry as a whole. No doubt that some of the people who developed genetically modified, herbicide-resistant crop strains thought they were feeding the world, all the while never realizing that their produce would contaminate the entire planet.

A hypnosis colleague, James M. Vera, author of the book *Hypnoketosis: Eat the Foods You Love and Lose Weight While You Sleep*, teaches his clients to shop the perimeter of the supermarket. In other words, avoid all the processed foods in the interior aisles. I love that strategy because it makes shopping simple. And in general, it is true. You are more likely to find real food on the supermarket's perimeter than inside the aisles. I often recommend Vera's book to my own clients.

I encourage my clients to read labels, including in the supermarket's dairy section, which is often a perimeter department. We learn to identify ingredients and avoid those that can cause difficulties. Shredded cheese usually has additives to stop it from caking. Yogurts may have the fat removed, and sugars or non-nutritive sweeteners added. Juices are pure sugar. American cheese is a *processed cheese*, meaning it is manufactured using more than one kind of cheese but may have other ingredients added. It's like the dairy version of a hot dog, *mostly* meat. Anything labeled *processed cheese food* is likely less than half cheese. Get into the habit of reading labels!

While I owe the ketogenic community a big thank you

for creating recipes with good macronutrient ratios, I have watched those keto cooks go to extraordinary lengths with extremely complicated recipes to pardon the expression, have their cake, and eat it, too. In my mind, non-nutritive sweeteners only extend the problem, the way nicotine gum or vaping becomes as addictive as smoking.

I can understand compensating in this way while we adjust to a new lifestyle. Consuming manufactured keto-friendly food, or food that is made at home from highly processed ingredients, is not eating real food and indicates a certain amount of unwillingness to change. I mentioned earlier how I tried lots of bread and pasta recipes because I didn't want to give those things up. Five stars for trying but most of those recipes were disappointing and expensive. I ended up with pricy ingredients in my pantry that I would never ever use again. While I didn't like the idea of giving up a plate of spaghetti, I later found ways of doing just that.

It took a while for me to be ready to say that certain foods just weren't worth eating. Determining that a food is not worth eating doesn't mean I can't eat it ever again. I can and may do so in very moderate quantities from time to time. After a while, products made mostly from grains or starchy vegetables no longer played a central role in my meal planning. I just don't think about them. I have other foods to think about, things that *are* worth eating.

As I grew to accept the changes I needed to make, I invented my own dishes. I invented a thing I call *pizzagna*. It's like lasagna but without the noodles. It consists of all the wonderful ingredients that one would put on top of a pizza. I use pizza sauce (homemade), good mozzarella and parmesan cheeses, pepperoni, or my pepperoni-flavored homemade sausage, olives, mushrooms, and green peppers. It takes almost no time to prepare. I just had to learn the hard way to bake in a parchment-lined pan and let it cool a bit before indulging. In effect, it's like a deep-dish Chicago-style pizza without the crust. I'll take *pizzagna* over pizza any day.

I did almost the same thing with nachos. Several kinds of cheese, salsa, jalapeno rings, meat, olives, and a moderate amount of beans melted together, topped with a sprinkling of cilantro. Missing the crunch of the tortilla chips, I eat my *nachogna* with some crunchy flax seed crackers. No, they are not the same as regular nachos. I happen to think they are better. After all, while playing the role of bulk on a plate of nachos, the chips come in second to the toppings.

I use mung bean sprouts instead of noodles in soup. I use partially dehydrated zucchini strips instead of regular lasagna noodles. I use zucchetti instead of spaghetti. The trick is to not cook the zucchetti noodles at all. Just top them with piping hot sauce and tuck in. You have to make them fresh. The frozen ones are apt to be disappointing. And I actually like all of these things more than relying on the processed grains that used to fill my plate.

Changing macros by reducing carbs will help anyone lose weight and may positively affect their blood glucose levels, but unless the changes are both sustainable and the person is eating healthy real food, the effects are likely to be mixed and temporary. What good is that? Eating keto-friendly cheese curls or keto-friendly peanut butter cups isn't changing the lifestyle that developed metabolic disease and created obesity and type 2 diabetes. Neither does a person's relationship with food change. All it does is get us to spend a lot more money and *deceive ourselves into thinking we don't really need to change.* We can just live our frustrated junk-food addicted lives and lose a little weight at the same time.

I had a potential client call me and ask about my program. As I described the program, she interrupted and informed me that she had "done keto" for a length of time, but all the weight came back when she stopped. Of course it did! *She* hadn't changed. She might have consumed better macros for a while, but her lifestyle and mindset had not changed. I tried to explain the difference between my program and what she had done on her own. But she was having none of it. What a tragedy!

In her defense, many people make the same mistake both with the ketogenic diet and intermittent fasting. She didn't want to hear it. It's all for the better on my end. I don't want to work with anyone who doesn't want to change. And I've dismissed several clients who refused to do so.

The same sort of thing happens with so-called vegetarians who fill their carts with processed pseudo meat products. They get to have their scruples and their burgers, too. I should know; I was one of them. I wanted to be a vegetarian, but I missed meat, so I developed tofu recipes, a myriad uses for textured vegetable protein, seitan (made from vital wheat gluten), Quorn® products. If I were still attempting that lifestyle, I would certainly be chowing down on Impossible™ Burgers that have become ubiquitous, all the while feeling good about my vegetarian ethics.

When vegetarians ask about my program, I ask them why they are vegetarian. If they believe it is a healthier lifestyle, I ask them if they are willing to consider other healthy options. If they tell me it's wrong to kill animals for food, my program is not for them. Protein sources for vegetarians also come with high carbohydrate content. You can't be a low-carb vegetarian without sacrificing protein or relying on processed food.

I've had clients who have clung tenaciously to their artificial sweeteners and wheat gluten bread. I do not force anyone to accept a change they aren't ready to make. It may take longer. The results may not be as dramatic. If they accept that *they* actually need to change, they may be ready later, in the future, to accept changes they won't consider today.

You must understand that for real change to happen, *you* have to change. Health won't come in a pill, and it won't come in a fad diet that eventually promises you can go back to eating the way you did before without consequences. It is often attributed to either Albert Einstein or Benjamin Franklin that the definition of insanity is doing the same thing over and over again and expecting different results. No matter who said it, it makes sense.

I've had clients discover they had changed without even realizing it. One client told me of a visit to his favorite pizza parlor, a place he had frequented so often they recognized him and knew him by name. As he bit into the pizza, it didn't taste right. He asked the person behind the counter if they had changed anything about the recipe, a different sauce or cheese or crust recipe. They assured him that nothing had changed since his last visit.

"As I sat there, I realized something. If the pizza hadn't changed, it must be that I had." He didn't finish the pizza.

Now there are many people who follow a ketogenic diet that focus on real food and don't fall into the keto krap trap. Those who embrace the world of real food lead happier, healthier lives. Those who cling to the keto krap will discover that their lives have not really benefited. They may have lost weight and even kept it off, but that processed pseudo food isn't healthy, in my opinion, and since they haven't changed inside, they are likely to go back to their old ways when they get tired of paying those premium prices.

I really think that deleting diabetes is like deleting a file on your computer. It doesn't disappear and can always be found again. So let's embrace change, a new, authentically fulfilling lifestyle that nurtures health, wellness, and happiness.

Chapter 8:
The Big Fat Scam

My biggest problem with the high-fat part of the low-carb and high-fat diet had two facets. The first was that I knew fat had twice the number of calories than either proteins or carbohydrates. I got over that pretty quickly simply by learning the simplified science of how the body processes macronutrients. Calories simply didn't matter the way I thought they did.

The bigger hurdle was the mental association between saturated fat, cholesterol, and cardiovascular disease. Remember Ancel Keys and the heart-health hypothesis? Like most people in society, I had taken the bait, hook, line, and sinker, as the cliche goes. The book that finally turned me around was *The Big Fat Surprise: Why Butter, Meat and*

Cheese Belong in a Healthy Diet by Nina Teicholz. She documented the unreliable science of Ancel Keys and the contradicting but better science of those who dared oppose him. As we know, Keys' propaganda won the battle for the American mind.

It has been drummed into our heads that saturated fat, animal fat, lard, bacon, egg yolks, etc. are bad and that polyunsaturated fats such as corn oil, vegetable oil, canola oil, rapeseed oil, soybean oil, and sunflower oil are good, mainly under the misconception that eating saturated fat causes heart disease. If you want to know the history in detail, I recommend Nina Teicholz's book, *The Big Fat Surprise*.

If you are anywhere near my age, you probably remember the back and forth about eggs and whether or not they are healthy. At one point, the recommended limit was set at only two whole eggs per week. As I read Teicholz's book, my thoughts harkened to the Noakes trial. This whole fat argument was ultimately about money and market share. The media circus that went back and forth, finally deciding on the lipid hypothesis as the one we would keep, was all about whose wallets would get the fattest. It seems that the current shift toward plant-based everything, which also happens to be processed food, is just another extension of that hypothesis.

Remember, I was a vegetarian for many years. Although I started eating meat again on my own, an influential book debunking many arguments in favor of vegetarianism and veganism is *The Vegetarian Myth*, by Lierre Keith. She comes off a little heavy-handed, but some might say the same thing about me. The book makes its point clearly: Monoculture industrial agriculture damages the planet more than humane animal husbandry, animals replenish the soil while industrial agriculture has to augment the soil with artificial chemicals and herbicides, and vegetarians are hungry nearly all the time. Keith's book is a challenging read for those who believe that a vegetarian or vegan lifestyle is healthier and better for the planet.

When I was watching the Noakes trial, the one part I had the most trouble embracing was the high-fat side of the low-carb and high-fat diet. As I learned about the importance of saturated fat in the absorption of many nutrients, I began looking at the supplements I was taking. The vitamins in gel caps were all encased in cheap vegetable oil, most often genetically modified. I was wasting my money on supplements to provide nutrients that my body wouldn't really absorb anyway because vegetable oils are not as efficient as saturated fats. You can eat all the nutrient-rich food and take all the supplements you want, but without a certain amount of saturated fat, many nutrients may be barely if at all absorbed by the body.

It was obvious to me that the promotion of polyunsaturated fats had more to do with wealth than health. You can't squeeze corn and get oil out. The abundance of subsidized grains produced by industrial monoculture farming created a need for innovative ways of using those products. George Washington Carver squeezed peanuts and got oil but intended the oil to be burned, not consumed. Other seed oils must be chemically extracted, thus altering their essential nature.

Polyunsaturated oils oxidize quickly, especially when heated, rendering them damaging and perhaps even toxic. Seed oil consumption has been linked to more than one symptomatic condition of metabolic disease, plays a role in inflammation, and is associated with DNA and central nervous system damage. In contrast, there is no evidence that saturated animal fat does anything of the sort. Despite these concerns, few nutritionists or physicians warn their patients off chemically extracted seed oils, but they do warn them off saturated fat.

Even the cholesterol scare seems to have been a victim of the heart health hypothesis. Many of the authors listed at the end of this book point out that high levels of LDL cholesterol actually have a positive effect when considering all-cause mortality. People, especially women, actually live longer.

Statins, the drugs used to reduce cholesterol come with many side effects. Given the assumption, and it is only an assumption, that high levels of cholesterol cause heart attacks, it is a tradeoff many doctors assume is worth making. The standard procedure to consider LDL levels of cholesterol warranting a statin prescription is just another example of treating a symptomatic condition without addressing the cause of what we now understand as metabolic disease.

While oxidation of polyunsaturated oils is one big problem, another is the excessive glycation of LDL cholesterol molecules. In other words, the excess glucose in our bloodstream alters (sugar coats) the LDL cholesterol molecules rendering them unrecognizable by the liver as something that needs to be cleansed from the system. What? The liver is responsible for controlling the levels of LDL cholesterol. Take care of your liver, and it will take care of you.

Again, the problem at the base of the issue is the excess carbohydrates are converted into glucose. The glycation of LDL cholesterol is yet another reason to cut back on those carbs.

The more I learn about this area of health research, the less I want anything to do with polyunsaturated oils. Granted, when I'm eating out, I don't have much choice in the oils the restaurant chooses to use, which is undoubtedly the cheapest they can get. I rarely choose to eat anything fried in a restaurant. I won't say I never eat it, but it is a rare occasion. Furthermore, because they are so cheap, those seed oils are added as ingredients into many processed foods, even the ones advertised as keto-friendly. For me, the presence of these oils on a list of ingredients is most often a deal-breaker when it comes to a buying decision.

I remember my father saving lard and bacon drippings in a can and using it to fry his eggs. Talk about a double whammy for the lipid hypothesis! Today, in honor of my father and my family's health, I've got a jar of bacon drippings in the fridge, which I use with frequency. Any time I might put oil in a pan, my choice is saturated fat. I don't really cook with olive oil, a monounsaturated fat, because it oxidizes. I use it mostly in salads or to top a vegetable dish *after* it has been cooked. At that, I use only extra virgin, cold-pressed olive oil.

If you are put off by pork for whatever reason, lamb fat, beef tallow, duck fat, or chicken fat will do the same job.

When I purchase chicken parts with the skin on, I cut up the skin and render the fat. The crispy, lightly salted skin is delicious, full of protein and no carbs, and the drippings saved in the fridge are wonderful for pan or stir-frying meat and vegetables.

But of course, I don't really want you to believe me. Do your research and make your own decisions. I stopped taking the statin my doctor prescribed, and every time I see him, he tries to get me to go back on it. I'll bet my refusal is clearly noted in my file. I don't mind. I've taken both responsibility and ownership of my health. My LDL cholesterol is a little high, but my triglycerides, which are more indicative of potential cardiovascular risks, are fine.

Chapter 9:
Reducing Carbohydrates &
Therapeutic Intermittent Fasting

———— ❦ ————

If we accept that metabolic disease occurs because consuming excess sugar and other carbohydrates triggers hyperinsulinemia, and if we understand that excess body fat is the body's way of coping with all that excess glucose, the solution is clear. Eat fewer carbohydrates and give the body enough time between meals so that it must begin to use its stored energy. It's that simple.

You may have heard the old adage, if you are in a hole and want to get out, the first thing you should do is stop digging. It should suffice to merely suggest that we make carbohydrates the smallest portion of our menu. That is easier said than done because of the way we have been trained to eat carbohydrates. I challenge you to go to any of your favorite restaurants and look for low-carb options. Go to any buffet or banquet and look at what is being served. The largest percentage of what is on offer consists of either pure carbohydrates or dishes bulked up by carbohydrates.

Americans worldwide are known for eating large portions. When we understand the role of carbohydrates in our standard diet, it's no mystery why that is true. Carbohydrates, being processed quickly by our body, cause hunger to resurface, sometimes before even finishing a meal. After all, there's always room for dessert.

I started my journey simply by cutting my carbohydrate portions in half and later half again. Within a couple of weeks, I was consuming less than 25% of the carbohydrates than before, even as a well-behaved type 2 diabetic. It was a decent plan at first because it was one that I could live with at the time. The thought of never ever eating another ear of corn, for example, was intolerable. Never again having any pasta or bread was inconceivable. If I had attempted that kind of change before I was emotionally ready for it, I would have given up and might well be injecting insulin today. So gradual change can be quite handy.

When I was eating only 25% of the carbohydrates, two things happened. The first was that my hunger changed. I wasn't as hungry as I had been before my journey began. I learned that when I consumed carbohydrates, feelings of hunger would return sooner than if I confined my plate to protein, fat, and vegetables. Vegetables make up the bulk on the plate, and the fat picks up the caloric values that keep my body functioning without going into starvation mode.

Of course, the added advantage of fat is that it signals feelings of satiety. Back in my carboholic life, I would feel hungry even if I felt full. I had no idea what being satisfied felt like until I felt overfull. I'm sure some people would have looked at me and thought I was a compulsive eater. Perhaps I was because continuing to eat when you know your stomach is full is a relatively good indication of compulsive eating behavior. But I want to make it clear that I really felt hungry, or at least I thought I felt hungry. Understanding and identifying the feeling of being satisfied is something I work on with my clients. It seems to be a common enough problem in both weight loss and diabetes control.

When I was a vegetarian, I was *always* hungry. And that feeling of being hungry even when the stomach is full is a kind of hunger triggered by even a slight drop in blood glucose levels. You can still have blood sugar levels through the roof and feel hungry because once the insulin kicks in, the associated drop in blood glucose seems to trigger feelings of hunger. Some people accustomed to high blood glucose levels actually feel symptoms of hypoglycemia (low blood sugar) when the actual glucose in their blood is well above the recognized levels for low blood sugar.

The second thing that happened when I was down to about 25% of my former carbohydrate consumption was that my enjoyment of them began to wane. The portions of those carbohydrates seemed so insignificant that it was no longer worth eating them, much less cooking them. I didn't need them. I no longer craved them. They began to seem pointless. I began to perceive them as worthless bulk on the plate. It became easier and more satisfying to simply not bother.

Sometimes, if carbohydrates were part of another dish, say noodles in soup, I found myself picking them out. They didn't add to my enjoyment of the soup. If picking them out was too difficult, I would try to eat around them or just not finish the bowl when the noodles became too prominent. The soup wasn't going to do much to my blood sugar levels, but the noodles or potatoes would. They didn't seem worth eating.

Today, I get most of my carbohydrates from the trace amounts found in above-ground vegetables. In my practice, I find that people who don't like vegetables most often simply don't know how to prepare them. And often enough, when I let them know they can use bacon fat or butter (never margarine) to prepare those vegetables, they visibly brighten.

The thing about a low-carb diet, especially one that encourages healthy fat, allows for really tasty vegetable dishes. Cream sauces made with heavy cream and butter instead of skim milk thickened with flour are absolutely indulgent. Vegetables sauteed in bacon fat or butter seasoned with onion, garlic, or a myriad of spices probably already in your kitchen are delightful.

If it's a texture issue, change the texture. Cook them longer or shorter or eat them raw if you prefer crunch to something softer. Puree them if you want a smooth texture. Vegetables in a soup made with good homemade bone broth can be pureed and made into a creamy soup with a stick blender and a bit of butter and cream. There is nothing better than cauliflower covered with a wonderful cheese sauce made from quality cheese, cream, a bit of bone broth, and butter.

A salad at the end of the meal is always a good choice. The vinegar aids in digestion, and it's different enough from the rest of the meal to constitute a good final course. I don't know why salad is served first as an appetizer in restaurants. Probably it's because they want you also to buy a dessert.

In my house, there are always nuts, olives, and cheese, and if at the end of the meal, we still want a bit more, we enjoy those. All contain fat and promote the feeling of being satisfied.

Cutting carbohydrates may seem difficult because they are everywhere and eating less and less of them limits our choices. You have to ignore the displays of candy and chips you encounter in the check-out line in virtually every store. When you walk by the bakery section in the supermarket, don't bother picking up bread or your favorite breakfast cereal that you no longer eat. Shopping and cooking become a whole new experience,

You can imagine looking at a menu in a restaurant and thinking, *There is nothing on this menu that is not packed with carbohydrates.* It happens a lot, and one gets either used to asking for substitutions or leaving half the food on the plate. Most restaurants will serve a burger without the bun, but choosing something to go along with that burger can be quite a challenge. Here in Pittsburgh, many salads come with french fries, not on the side but in the salad, and often with additional croutons!

Life gets surprisingly easy once you get used to weeding

out the carbs. You can ignore 90% of the supermarket. Even if you walk down all the aisles, you can walk pretty quickly. Shopping is quick and easy. You become better at picking out meat and more adventurous about vegetables.

You'll also create a mental plan for most of the restaurants you frequent. Some of them aren't worth going to but having figured out the menus for those you really like, and you won't even have to look at the menu. Most restaurants can accommodate you to some degree.

I don't eat out in restaurants often, but when I do, I can find something I can eat. After I achieved my goal of deleting my diabetes, I have taken a rare liberty here and there. I might eat a couple of onion rings, a piece of fried chicken, or a piece of batter-dipped fish. These are bad choices for both the carbohydrates and the oil in which they are fried. Remember that you will have wiggle room, but you won't want to wiggle as much as you think you might.

Chapter 10:
Therapeutic Intermittent Fasting

W hat many people think of as intermittent fasting isn't intermittent at all. People do the easy part of fasting by increasing the time between their bite of food in the evening and their first bite in the morning, usually by eating their first meal later in the day. I call this fast the *natural* fast. Since most of their fasting time is spent sleeping, it's easy, but it's not intermittent. It's useful, but not useful enough.

Increasing the natural fast is important because it gives our body time to use up much of the ready glucose in the blood and begin the process of gluconeogenesis. This is what is supposed to happen during the natural fast. More than 80% of the American population suffers from at least some degree of metabolic disease, having one or more of the symptomatic conditions. In a healthy person, it can take up to 24 hours of fasting to deplete glycogen. In an insulin-resistant person, we might expect it to be even longer.

Within the timeframe of the natural fast, even when we extend it to 16 to 18 hours, we cannot expect to deplete glycogen fully. Therefore, once we have grown accustomed to a longer natural fast, we can then begin to think about therapeutic intermittent fasting. I teach my clients that a therapeutic intermittent fast is one that lasts at least 24 hours. Even then, we might not fully deplete glycogen stores in the beginning.

Here's some good news. If our natural fast routine is long enough to start using up glycogen stores, the cells in our body may become less resistant to insulin, especially if we are being active during our waking hours. The more active we are, the more our cells need glucose. As we use the glucose in our blood, the liver recognizes the reduction and, as long as we haven't eaten anything, begins to burn glycogen. Now you know why a reduced carbohydrate diet is so effective and why combining with therapeutic intermittent fasting is so powerful.

The good news is that once we are in ketosis, it can take up to 48 hours to replenish those glycogen stores giving us more time to burn fat.

At least for the first year or two, we have to factor in the lag time created because of insulin resistance. I admit I have watched very complicated scientific presentations on the nature of insulin resistance, but for me to relate that here with any degree of accuracy would be an exercise in absurdity. I'd surely get it wrong, so let me explain it in the way I understand it, and you decide if my explanation works for you.

It's not as simple as the cells are full and don't want or need any more glucose. Think of that parent spoon-feeding their baby, continuing to shovel in spoonfuls of food, and the baby keeps turning away because it isn't hungry. Overfull cells are only part of insulin resistance.

Those cells have been so full for so long that they have built up defensive barriers to prevent the next insult of glucose.

Think of blowing up a balloon. The fuller the balloon gets, the more blowing pressure you need to use. That is one aspect. The second aspect happens when you begin to feel uncomfortable blowing up the balloon because you are afraid it will burst in your face. It is as if the balloon itself is communicating to you through its resistance, suggesting that you are going too far. Not only do the cells need to be willing to accept more glucose when they need it, but they also need to trust that they won't be barraged again with copious amounts of excess glucose. And that takes a complete lifestyle change. Both aspects need to be addressed.

Increasing the natural fast to between 16 to 18 hours every day allows our body to begin those important first aspect processes. In that time frame, we are well into our glycogen stores, and the cells of our body are accepting glucose because they need it. Making that natural fast consistent gives them the confidence to be a little more trusting.

People who think that extending the natural fast is intermittent fasting are merely eating less. Many try to combine extending the natural fast with a reduced-calorie diet. Of course, they lose weight. Any diet will work for a while. But their body wants homeostasis, that is, to stay the same. When they do this, they are converting a fasting regime into a calorie-restrictive diet that causes their metabolism to go into starvation mode and actually slows down.

This shift in metabolic rate is what is essentially wrong and even dangerous about a calorie-restricted diet, especially one that demands physical exertion, ostensibly in the name of burning more calories. When the desired weight is achieved, the habits loosen, and the calories go up. The body's first priority is to maintain the reduced metabolic rate while it restocks the level of energy reserves it thinks is normal for the dieter. The weight comes back.

Someone who has extended their natural fast from 10 to 16 hours will lose a bit of weight, but as soon as the body considers that pattern to be normal, the weight may well return. When I'm working with clients, we gradually increase the natural fast until we reach a standard 16 to 18 hours, leaving an eating window of 6 or 8 hours. We understand that there may be times when we occasionally have a shorter fast, and after we reach our goal, we might loosen up a bit, but that standard natural fast, which allows for an eight-hour eating window, becomes our new normal.

Once that natural fast pattern is established, we introduce longer fasting periods *intermittently*. I emphasize the intermittent nature because we don't want to develop patterns that the body thinks are becoming normal before we reach our goals, whatever they may be.

Our first intermittent fasting attempt will be a 24-hour fast.

Breakfast to breakfast, lunch to lunch, or dinner to dinner. While on my program, we try several different fasting patterns that we apply intermittently. Prescriptively in the program, we don't go beyond 36 hours of fasting, but many clients choose to do longer fasts of 48 or 72 hours. The longest I've personally fasted was for five days, and I felt great.

While on a fast, we consume nothing that might stimulate blood glucose or insulin. Water and black unsweetened tea or coffee, herbal teas included, are the most common choices. Our bodies will be producing glucose and in time, ketones, and the longer we go without eating, the more stored energy is used. When we eat the first meal after a fast, we plan a meal without carbohydrates just to prolong the effects of the longer fast as long as possible.

The point of the longer fasts is to deplete glycogen stores and have the liver access body fat as a fuel source. Once glycogen stores have been depleted, it can take up to 48 hours to replenish them. If we maintain a low carbohydrate diet, replenishing glycogen may take perhaps even longer simply because the amount of glucose is limited. Given that condition, we can remain in ketosis, often utilizing both ketones and glucose for quite a long time. This is one of the reasons why some people on the ketogenic diet count carbs so diligently. The obvious advantage of remaining in ketosis is that fat remains a constant fuel source.

I hope you now see why longer fasts are necessary. We aren't working for a quick and likely temporary change in our bodies. On a diet, we may lose weight temporarily, but the body doesn't recognize the permanence of the change. We want to train our bodies to change their default settings. For years and years, we've been building up surplus glucose and body fat. It's time to reverse the process and allow the body to finally use and enjoy the stored energy it's been squirreling away for decades. It's kind of a reward vacation for our bodily functions. Apart from some physical damage, the body *wants* to do this.

Also, along the way, you may discover that your most comfortable lifestyle doesn't depend on comfort foods and desserts. As the body changes, the way it uses energy also changes. You will discover that you have more energy. You will sleep better. Your libido might increase. And what you think of as pleasant or fun can change. As your body adjusts, other symptomatic conditions of metabolic disease will likely change. You may, for example, find out your blood pressure medication is too strong.

Regarding blood pressure, I discovered as I became more active that I would feel light-headed, particularly on days when I was doing a lot of activities, working hard out in the yard, or taking on projects around the house that demanded significant time. I discovered that my blood pressure medication was too strong. Using my home blood pressure cuff, I could see that my blood pressure numbers were changing. My doctor agreed to cut down on my medication when I discussed it. He might have attributed the change to weight loss. Perhaps it was. All I know is that the prescription changed.

The first 24-hour fasting period can be a stretch. Often fasting beyond the average natural fasting time, 16 to 18 hours, can trigger almost compulsive thoughts of eating even though the body and our blood glucose levels may be fine. It is critical that during your longer fasts, you keep an eye on your blood glucose levels if you are still taking medications.

Don't be distracted by the last sentence. I am not suggesting that you should or should not still be taking medications for diabetes. I've worked with enough people to know that when it becomes appropriate to change the dosage of a diabetes medication is as individual as a fingerprint. For me, it was a matter of weeks. For others, it may be a matter of months. I strongly encourage you to discuss dosage-changing procedures with your doctor. If your doctor is at all aware of the impact of a low-carb and intermittent fasting regimen, they will know this is important. If they are unwilling to discuss this with you, consider getting a second opinion. I've had clients tell me about the different reactions of their doctors. They range from collegial and supportive to outright irrational.

You have to prepare for that first 24-hour fast.

- Choose a day when you expect to be reasonably busy.

- Test your blood glucose frequently, especially at and after your natural fasting time limit. If you are still taking medications that might cause low blood sugar levels, keep handy some juice, honey sticks, or some other rapid form of glucose if you notice the symptoms of low blood sugar.

- Plan what you will eat to break your fast so that you aren't just grabbing any food available once you reach the time.

Often people struggle with the last few hours of their first 24-hour fast, mostly because their body is used to eating something at that time. If you find yourself compulsively looking at the clock and counting the hours and minutes until you can eat, take a moment and breathe and relax. Observe the feelings of hunger and thank your body for taking care of you. It sounds crazy but tell your body, out loud if you can without embarrassment, that you will eat soon, sometime after whatever hour your fast ends. It's incredible, but it seems to work.

On your first attempt, you may also want to have handy a cup of good quality bone broth. If you become irrationally hungry, look at the clock, and tell yourself that you'll have that cup of broth in an hour. If when you reach that time, you think you can't make it to 24 hours, heat and mindfully sip that broth. It will work wonders.

Technically, bone broth will break your fast but only for a short while. Bone broth is not something we normally consume during a fast. Our goal is to gently get used to longer fasts. Believe me when I tell you that you will discover and learn the tricks that work best for you along the way.

If you are going to use a commercial bone broth, read the labels, make sure there aren't carbohydrates in it, and that it isn't filled with chemicals and ingredients that your body won't recognize as food. It should be almost jelly-like to provide collagen and the nutrition of the bones. Commercial bone broth is rarely as good as you can make at home. I don't recommend any commercial bone broth.

The recipe and instructions for the best homemade bone broth are simple, but it is a three-day process. Save the bones from any meal. Cooked bones are better. I save them all: chicken carcasses, bones from pork, beef, and lamb. Lightly rinse them and freeze them until you can loosely fill your crock pot. Also, wash your vegetables before peeling them; save the peels, onion skins, celery trimmings, garlic skins, and any tops and tails of above-ground veggies. Freeze them in a separate container.

On day one, fill your crockpot with the frozen bones. Add a small handful of a good-quality salt. I use Himalayan pink salt, but kosher salt is also good—just not salts with some additive that prevents caking. Fill the crockpot with filtered water. Set the crockpot to low and wait until the next day.

On day two, strain the broth through a colander. Don't worry about any bits that get through the colander. Set aside this broth and put it in the refrigerator when it's cool enough. From the colander, take only the bones. If bits of meat have come off those bones, we don't want them in the crockpot again. As you are picking the bones, try to break them to reveal the marrow. If you are using chicken or turkey bones, the knuckles should break off fairly easily. Other bones usually already show some marrow. Fill the crockpot with filtered water, another small handful of salt, and set it to low. Wait until tomorrow.

On day three, strain the broth through a colander and toss out the bones. Put it with the first batch of broth. That first batch should look like jelly with a layer of fat on the top. Do not trim the fat. It's good for you!

Now get your veggies and put them in the pot with another bit of salt. Add any aromatics, spices, or herbs you want. I usually put in a bay leaf, a bit of garlic, and parsley. Fill the pot with filtered water, set on low, and wait. Eight or nine hours is usually enough. The water is boiling, the veggies are soft, and you can smell good soup. Strain the soup through a colander. Again, don't worry about any little bits that get through.

Combine all three batches together and heat until it's all well mixed and all the fat is melted. You can put this broth into containers and freeze it. Choose containers that are half-portion size because the broth is strong enough to dilute it when you are ready. I store it in half-cup sizes and pint sizes. The half-cup size will make a cup of bone broth, or I can add things to make a single serving of soup. The pint sizes are for when I am making soup for two.

OMAD stands for <u>o</u>ne <u>m</u>eal <u>a</u> <u>d</u>ay. In my book, OMAD is the smallest fasting time frame for therapeutic intermittent fasting. Once you've done one, you know you can and you will. The next step is simple. Do it several times a week, always following the planning steps. Some people stop here. They might OMAD fast three times a week or do it every day. The important thing to remember is if you are eating one meal a day, that meal should contain enough nutrition to sustain your health and enough calories to convince your body you are not starving or depriving yourself. It should be a full meal, but OMAD is not a license to pig out on carbs. The low-carb element must remain.

Most of us, however, want to move on to even longer fasts because, after a while, they almost become addictive. It is freeing to know that you don't have to eat just because your stomach growls or simply because there is something tasty available. When I'm traveling, I always have the option to not eat, especially if there is nothing worth eating available. Because I am no stranger to fasting, the lack of healthy real food isn't a problem, even for several days. I just don't worry about it.

After you do several OMADs a week, try a new stretch. Do three OMADs in a row, staggering the meals you consume. Consider breakfast to lunch, lunch to dinner, and finally dinner to dinner. The last one is the easiest, of course, but none of them should be too difficult for an experienced faster like you.

The next step is a 36-hour fast. If you haven't been in ketosis yet, you will be on a fast for this duration. Get those test strips ready! I find a dinner to breakfast pattern the easiest to manage. On the day prior to your first 36-hour fast, eat a good, low-carb dinner. Get a good night's sleep. Fast the entire day and go to bed without your supper. You can break your fast the next morning, or if you aren't hungry because you are used to not eating breakfast, you can fast longer and wait until lunch. You don't have to fast in 12-hour increments.

In my first book, *The Hypnofasting Program Guide: A Practical Plan to Lose Weight and Control Type 2 Diabetes*, I described my favorite fasting pattern.

You start with a 36-hour fast. Then have an eating day with an eating window of perhaps six hours or two meals. Then do an OMAD, with a meal following. Then another 36-hour fast.

Especially in the beginning, longer fasts can have unique challenges. I've prepared a more extensive list of suggestions, some of which are the same as the ones for your first OMAD.

1) Plan your fast ahead of time from beginning to end. Psychologically prepare yourself to begin your fast at a particular time on a day and date that is convenient. Choose a time period that is unlikely to include undue stress but during which you can keep yourself occupied.

2) The first 48 hours, particularly the second day, can be the most difficult for many people. For me, it depends on what is happening on which day. If either day is unexpectedly stressful, I find I think of food more often because my brain is trying to escape the stress. After all, that's what stress eating is all about.

3) Consume no obvious carbohydrates the day before beginning your fast. Consume only fats and proteins as much as possible.

4) Testing Blood Glucose: If you are still taking diabetes medications, you will need to test your blood glucose levels regularly, especially if your medications might contribute to low blood sugar. You won't be eating, and your medications are designed to compensate for food. Keep fruit juice or honey sticks handy in case you experience low blood sugar.

5) If you test for ketones, do so the morning of the first full day of your fast and then intermittently throughout the fasting period. (It really helps to see your progress.)

6) Do **not** weigh yourself. Your weight will fluctuate during and after the fast. That is actually a good

thing. It means your body is figuring out what you did. In any case, weight is not a good short-term measure of progress. Even if it appears you have regained the weight you lost on a longer fast, you still have made progress toward restoring your health by putting a dent into glycogen and burning some fat.

7) Stay hydrated. Drink only water during your fasting period. Other possibilities include black unsweetened coffee or tea—no creamers or artificial sweeteners. Herbal and green teas are also fine, as are sips of pickle juice (check for any sugar) and, of course, diluted apple cider vinegar. You might also consider a dash of salt once in a while, especially if you have stopped consuming processed foods, our biggest salt source. Without processed food, many of us actually need to add salt to our diet.

8) In choosing the length of your fast, calculate the end day, date, and time of your fast and tell yourself that you *can* (not *will*) eat *after* (not *at*) that hour. This psychological trick leaves the plan open to extending the fasting period if you need or choose to. It also ensures that you aren't irrationally ravenous when the fast is coming to an end. Remind yourself of this goal when your body signals hunger. Just breathe and let it know that you plan to eat again after that time.

9) Watch your internal monologue. Telling yourself that you are hungry, or worse, *starving*, will only make the experience more intolerable. This internal conversation is a kind of -hypnosis that can actually

cause your body to react as if you really are starving. So perish the thought, literally. Stop it in its tracks. When you experience hunger, observe it, don't judge it as good or bad. Find it in your body and watch it instead of trying to get away from it. It seems unpleasant, but when it's observed, it is less so. It's just your body reacting to a temporary condition.

10) Set up a strategy for managing coercive hunger. That is, plan ahead in the event of intolerable suffering. Suffering is a highly personal perception, and indeed, a fair amount of suffering happens in the brain, not the body. If you have ever forgotten to eat, it was because your brain was engaged in another task. What some people consider uncomfortable, others might consider insufferable. Plan and provide a temporary respite that will not greatly increase your blood glucose or stimulate insulin. Consider a beverage you can mindfully sip. A hot beverage seems to work for some people better than a cold one, so you are likely already drinking something. For moments that seem a bit out of hand, consider coffee with heavy cream, coconut oil or MCT oil, or good-quality bone broth. Because hunger is curbed using fat and fat stimulates insulin the least, we choose drinks that are high in fat. They will break your fast but for a minimal time. Here's a strategy for dealing with sketchy moments:

1) When you notice that you can't seem to distract your mind from feeling hunger, look at the clock and choose a time at least an hour later, telling yourself that you **can** (not *will*) partake **after** (not

at) that time.

2) Plan your beverage. Make sure you have the ingredients handy, and the means to produce the beverage should you need it.

3) When the time arrives, if the crisis has passed, don't partake. Just continue. If the crisis has not passed, drink a glass of filtered water and then intentionally and mindfully partake of your beverage in sips. Do NOTHING else while partaking. Focus your attention on your sips.

11) Be cautious of leisure time, especially if you were someone who used to eat for emotional reasons. You can try setting an occupational goal for the duration of your fast. If it is an active goal, all the better. Cleaning out the garage, fixing that loose step, weeding the garden, trimming the hedge are goals that might be fit into the timeframe of a longer fast. Having a more immediate goal helps because fasting has a long-term, not a short-term goal. In these days of immediate gratification, long-term goals seem less urgent and less important. Many lose their tenacity in working toward long-term goals when confronted with what seems like an immediate need.

12) A prolonged fast is not the time to collect recipes or watch food videos. You'll know how much food occupies your mind by the things social media suggests to you. If YouTube sends you lots of cooking videos, or you see advertisements for foods, restaurants, kitchen gadgets, or utensils on other sites, you've been

shopping for those things.

13) If you find yourself writhing in hunger, clutching your stomach, and you can't stop thinking about food, look at the clock and tell yourself you can eat after an hour. If the crisis hasn't passed, for heaven's sake, eat something. A hardboiled egg might get you through so you can go back to your fast. The fast will be broken, but it's better than all that internal conflict. If you can't just go back to your fast, end your fast there and try again later. Believe me, it gets easier with experience.

I gave myself three years to address my type 2 diabetes, and nearly a year ago now, a test result indicated that I was no longer insulin resistant. I considered that moment the one in which I achieved my objective. I moved into maintenance mode. My natural fast has relaxed a bit. It usually falls between 14 and 16 hours. I still do longer fasts but much less frequently.

I'll do an OMAD or two every couple of weeks, just to keep in the game. If I notice changes like gaining a few pounds, indulging in snacks too often, or noticing old habits starting to creep back in, I'll do a longer, more extended pattern of several days. I've fasted once for five days and might think about doing a fast like that once or twice a year. I still have a bit of extra weight around the middle. I haven't decided yet whether or not to tackle it. The point is that this is my new lifestyle. I eat low carb with occasional increases that knock me out of ketosis enough to make me want to do a longer fast. This new no-longer-diabetic lifestyle is one I plan on keeping forever.

If you decide to delete your own diabetes, I am convinced

that combining a reduced carbohydrate diet with therapeutic intermittent fasting will allow your body to heal itself. How quickly the changes happen depends on how aggressively you pursue them and how much damage has already been done to your body by type 2 diabetes. How sustainable those changes are depends on how much you change from the inside out and your commitment to keeping those changes long enough for them to become part of your normal life.

There is, however, one thing you can do to speed up the process without risk and have some fun doing it. That is the subject of the next chapter.

Chapter 11:
The Dreaded E-word

❦

For many people, exercise is a dirty word. Most people think they need to exercise more, and some attempt to do so. They buy exercise equipment for their home. They join gyms with the best of intentions. They buy workout clothing, hoping to be inspired to wear it.

There are many reasons why our commitment to exercising rarely lasts long enough to make a difference. Some of them are obvious, others not so much.

On the practical side of things, a commitment to exercise adds another item to our to-do list. Most people don't really have that kind of room in their schedule. You might, for example, factor in an hour workout at the gym but fail to consider the time going and coming back, the time changing clothes, showering, laundering workout clothes, and packing or unpacking your workout bag. All of these things seem insignificant, but they add up, and if, for any reason at the gym, a person has to wait for something, a piece of equipment to come available, or a class to start, it becomes very time-consuming indeed. It is difficult to make room for those potential time-draining activities. Life gets in the way.

Often a person's reason for wanting to exercise comes from a negative emotion. We might say we want to lose weight, be more fit, be healthier, or be more attractive. Those sound like positive reasons, but they often spring from a deep dissatisfaction with who we are or how our lives have turned out. What we mean is we are unhappy being fat and out of shape, unhealthy, and unattractive. Those negative motivations may well be enough to get someone to sign a contract at a gym, but those motivations, those thoughts and emotions, are essentially soul-destroying. We need to love ourselves enough to want the best for ourselves.

Let's face it, exercise is unpleasant. Very few people actually enjoy exercise. The next time you tour a gym, look at the faces of the people who are there and count how many are smiling. They may enjoy particular activities but exercising for the sake of exercising is unappealing to most people. People who are successful in developing a fit lifestyle actually like the activities they choose to engage in.

Inertia is a powerful force. It's difficult to break any pattern of behavior. Going from a more sedentary lifestyle to a more active one is a big challenge, especially when we expect to live up to dramatic and radical changes straight away. We want results and are willing to pay for them, but when those results require more than money, many of us lose our commitment and motivation.

Exercise is artificial. It's not real. It is a contrived activity. Running on a treadmill doesn't get you anywhere. Running on a street might get you somewhere, but you aren't really going anywhere when you are running just to run. Exercise equipment has come a long way since people did basic circuit training but even a workout on the most interactive equipment, despite maps, screens of scenery, and coaching voices, is still artificial.

Many people see exercise as a form of punishment or payback for the excesses of life. They need to work off that donut, pizza, or fries they feel guilty about eating. For some, going to a gym is like turning themselves in to the police for having committed a crime.

And most of all, exercise doesn't work, at least not in the way we think it should. Doing half an hour on an elliptical machine is pointless if, after your workout, nothing changes especially if you stop for a smoothie on your way out of the gym.

Exercising to lose weight simply doesn't work. Your body acclimates to your general activity levels and treats spurts of activity as anomalies. Unless you work out at the gym consistently, regularly, and always trying to do more, your body may treat those rare workouts as sporadic and merely reset back to the old standard.

The ineffectiveness of exercise to lose weight should have

been obvious years ago. Back in the 1990s, when I was going to the gym semi-regularly, before choosing to focus on swimming in the early 2000s, after half an hour of using a treadmill or a stationary bike, the screen would advise me how many calories I had burned. Considering that the milk in my morning coffee had likely packed on more calories than I had just burned, that exercise was futile. So eventually, I stopped going, felt guilty for not going, and continued to pay for my membership because of the guilt and telling myself I'd start again, perhaps tomorrow—a complete waste of time, money, and mental energy that went on for years.

While regular exercise can help lift depression, it won't do much for your self-esteem. Even if you achieved a gym body, your mindset will cause you to look for other reasons you shouldn't like yourself. Loving and caring about yourself has to work its magic from the inside out.

Everyone seems to understand that loving and accepting themselves is a critical element of a happy life, but few people know how to go about actually doing that. In fact, I'd bet that many people reading this book might be embarking on that very journey as they read. Are you feeling better about yourself just reading this book? I hope so but if not, know that there is help. Counseling can help, but often self-love and self-esteem are not elements of mental illness. They are an unconscious response to conditions and circumstances that made us think that something was wrong and that, for some reason, we were different from other people. That concept moves people in the direction of blaming themselves, and if the blame falls on them, they think they have a logical reason to dislike themselves. That is the fundamental reason people try to make changes. They want to fix themselves so that the blame no longer falls on them.

In the context of this book, I can assure you that you are not overweight because you lack discipline or willpower. I can assure you that you are not diabetic because you are fat and lack discipline or willpower. You are not to be blamed for living in a society that has propagandized the concepts of a high-carbohydrate and low-fat diet on you and most effectively on your doctors, your nutritionists, and even your endocrinologists, who should all know better.

If we are going to use activity to increase our health and wellness, we've got to find the right motivation so that we engage in the activity regularly and consistently. Let's stop calling it exercise, anyway. That word carries too much emotional baggage. Instead of exercising more, let's say we want to increase our activity levels. I know that sounds boring, but increasing activity is a lot easier and way more effective than exercising.

Before we really get into it, let's get something straight: Exercise does not burn fat unless the body is already in fat-burning mode, that is, ketosis. The amount of calories burned in exercise is really subject to the fuel your body is using at the time. In any case, the ratio of exercise to food consumed, that is, calories-in and calories-out, is not direct. No matter how active you are, you can't keep up with the calories-in, calories-out paradigm. Calories are a measure of heat. We might get hot and sweaty while we work out, but when we lose weight, it doesn't disappear into heat. It just doesn't work that way.

When soda pop manufacturers suggest that calories are calories, it is a scam to convince you that sugar calories are the same as real food calories. They are not. All that misinformation does is help you justify buying and drinking sugary drinks because you think that with a little discipline and a bit more willpower, you burn them off at the gym or on the playing field. Even sports drinks get you to buy into that line. By now, you should be able to recognize why the claim is not true. If not, Gary Taubes, in his book, *Good Calories Bad Calories*, does an excellent job of explaining how and why a calorie is not just a calorie. Calories are not created equal and in terms of deleting diabetes, forgetting about calories altogether is by far a positive step.

Movement, of which "exercise" is just one kind, is not about using up calories but rather glucose. Get that into your head now: It's not about calories or burning fat. It is primarily about using glucose. Metabolic disease, hyperinsulinemia, and insulin resistance are the result of excess amounts of glucose in our blood, which is a dietary issue. Consuming copious amounts of carbohydrates generates all that excess glucose.

What matters is that when we increase our activity, our muscles, our cells need to use the glucose that is already stored in them. The more active we are, the more glucose they need to function properly and the more they use.

The connection between general activity levels and insulin resistance might already be obvious to you. If it isn't, let me make it clear. If we increase our activity levels, the cells of our body use the glucose stored in them. As they need to replace that glucose, they become more willing to accept glucose from the bloodstream. The more consistent we are with activity levels, the more the cells get used to accepting and using new supplies of glucose. That is the opposite of insulin resistance.

Now, let's explore the connection to weight loss. If our cells accept more glucose because their internal supplies are low, then the amount of excess glucose in our bloodstream diminishes. If there is little to no excess glucose in our blood, very little of it is sent to the liver for storage either as glycogen or body fat. In fact, the liver does what it wants to do. It *accesses* glycogen and fat and converts them into usable energy, glucose through gluconeogenesis, or ketones through ketosis.

If we are going to change our lifestyle to one that no longer accommodates type 2 diabetes, we don't need to *exercise* for half an hour three times a week. We need to *become* more active every day. We need to teach our bodies a new way of living and do it long enough that it becomes our new normal way of life.

We will never become more active people if we hate or resent the activity we are trying to adopt. The good news is that *any* activity we engage in will require the use of glucose. Indeed, our bodies use glucose all the time, even when we sleep. Our brains alone use around 20% of the glucose our bodies require. If we are consuming extra glucose-generating foods, like carbohydrates, it's all excess, no matter how much insulin you are injecting into your body. All the excess goes to create fat.

Activity is just another way of using glucose, but it is one that we can actually control. Moving requires energy. Whether we are parking in a more distant space, choosing to take the stairs instead of the elevator, cleaning out a closet, doing yard work, or washing the car by hand instead of driving through a carwash. In other words, any way we can increase our activity level will count. We need to just get up and move.

We don't have to jump into an exhausting workout to make a difference. The Chinese philosopher Lao Tzu is credited with the adage, "The journey of a thousand miles begins with one step." So let's start the first step.

There is probably a pedometer app on your phone. If there isn't one already, you can get one for free. Your phone already knows exactly where you are, so what actual privacy might you be sacrificing with a free pedometer app? You might have to watch a few commercials once in a while, but who cares? If you want to buy one, go ahead. It might save you the commercials, but the cloud already knows where you are when you are there.

You probably already keep your phone with you throughout the day. Look at your step count at the end of each day to see how many steps the pedometer counted for you. It doesn't even matter if it's accurate to your real steps. It counts motion, and that is what matters to us. You don't even have to go after the recommended 10,000 steps per day. Just see how much your phone thinks you are walking.

Once you have an idea of your normal activity levels, start looking for tiny, inconsequential ways of increasing your movement. Choose ways of just doing a little more at a time whenever you can. You'll know you are succeeding by looking at that step count each day. Just strive to do more tomorrow than today. Even one more step is still more. Make it a game. You'd be surprised how motivating a game can be. Of course, there will be days when you don't quite make it, especially if the day before was unusually active. You can easily recognize such overactive days and discount them. We don't want to discourage ourselves. Day by day, you'll feel better and more confident.

Eventually, when you are accustomed to moving more, you'll look to change your activity in different ways. Here's a tip from one of my clients. She chose to use a portion of her lunch break to walk around the parking lot of her office complex. The first day, she walked the perimeter of the lot just once. As she felt better about walking, she started getting creative. One lap turned to two, two laps into three, then laps turned to walking patterns between the parked spaces. She had fun.

One day she realized that when she listened to music while walking, she walked in pace with the music. For a nice brisk walk, she recommended disco, particularly the song, *Staying Alive* by the Bee Gees, the same song they say you should use when performing CPR. "By deleting my diabetes, I'm really doing it," she said. "I'm staying alive!"

I know this take on activity might sound ridiculous to you, but that is only because, in the back of your mind, you are still thinking about burning calories. Stop that! We aren't burning calories. Our cells are using glucose. We're not doing this to lose weight but to allow our bodies to function properly, to heal and reverse insulin resistance. That's the big news of the day!

I want to tell you a story about my own experience with walking. In the first years of my journey, I totaled my car. It was a stupid accident. No one was hurt, thank heavens.

I didn't have enough money to buy the car I really

wanted. I didn't want the cars I could afford, and I didn't want to incur debt for the next five years to get a payment that made financial sense to my budget. After burdening my husband, friends, and officemates for rides while I shopped for a car, I finally came to terms with reality. I'd be riding the bus until the car I wanted became affordable to me.

At the time, I rented two offices in health centers, one to the north and another to the south of the city. Driving to either took about 15 minutes, but by bus, it could be upwards of 2 hours plus. Both commutes required two buses with a transfer in downtown Pittsburgh. The commute to either office would be about an hour and a half with good connections, more than two hours if I had to wait for the next connecting bus. I didn't really mind riding the bus. I could listen to recorded books and relax to and from work. But four hours on the bus took up a big chunk of my working day.

Add to that time, the long walk from my home to my nearest bus stop took me at least 20 minutes. Pittsburgh is in the foothills of the Allegheny Mountains. While the downtown area is fairly flat, the surrounding boroughs are a different story. We have steep hills, and there are long flights of city sidewalk stairs. Some houses do not have direct street access. The only way to get to them is via city stairs. People who aren't from Pittsburgh find these steps quaint and interesting. Walking Pittsburghers (yes, that is what we call ourselves) find them indispensable time savers.

My 20-minute walk *to* the bus stop was all downhill. It included three flights of city stairs that totaled 120 individual steps. I counted them more than once. Coming home, the walk was all uphill. It took twice as long, and required breath-catching rests on landings and between flights of steps. My four hours on the bus were really closer to five if I included the walk.

One day, my first bus was running a few minutes late, and as we approached the downtown bus stop where I was to transfer, I saw my connecting bus arriving.

If I missed that bus, I'd have to wait another half an hour for the next one. Without thinking, I rushed off the first bus and ran a full city block in order to catch that connection. I didn't even think about it until after I was seated on the second bus. *I ran. I actually ran. I wasn't even breathless, and I ran a whole block!* That may seem insignificant to some of you, but to me, that was nothing short of a miracle. I was nearly 60 years old, and I hadn't run anywhere for any reason in probably 30 years!

I had a kind of storm in my mind. How did that happen? Certainly, by that time, I had lost a considerable amount of weight, and I required fewer rests on those stairs coming home. Even my time had improved. I had cut five minutes off the downhill walk and about 15 minutes off the walk from the bus stop home.

It's simple to increase activity levels without much exertion. Once your mind gets used to the idea that you aren't burning calories, any movement counts. Once you get used to the process, it will cease to be an effort. You'll just do it. In fact, you won't be pushing your body much, and after a while, your body will begin to push you. You'll have more energy and won't feel like sitting around all the time. You'll have more get up and go because you actually want to get up and go.

When this happens, start looking for fun things to do. Most people who have led sedentary lives often do not know where to even begin looking for fun activities. You might try some of the activities you used to enjoy as a younger, more active person. It is a good place to start, but you might also be disappointed in the quality of performance you feel you've lost over the years. It will come back. You simply haven't used those muscles and the corresponding brain circuitry for a while. You haven't completely lost the ability, but you might need to dust away some cobwebs.

Finding prosocial activities helps. Classes, bowling leagues, volunteering at the local food bank or thrift store or getting a part-time job are just a few activities to consider.

Perhaps there is something you always wanted to try like white water rafting or learning to kayak. If you don't have something like that, before joining a gym or hiring a private trainer, consider trying something completely new and different. Your local community college probably has adult learning classes fairly inexpensively. Many of them require moving around. You could learn to weld, fix cars, or even learn to cook. I guarantee in a cooking class, you are on your feet walking around most of the time.

Many local businesses, even gyms, offer free or low-cost introductory visitor passes to classes and lessons such as spin, Zumba, dance, yoga, tai chi, or other martial arts. You never know if you will like it, and a free lesson is risk-free. All it will cost you is listening to a sales pitch. If you hated the class, don't buy it. If you think you might like it, give it a try.

You might also look up hiking trails and groups that walk

them in your area. We have a rails-to-trails program in Pittsburgh that converts disused railroad passages to walking paths. The inclines are not steep, and the walks are pleasant. I've walked over 30 miles of those trails around Pittsburgh and never got bored because the trail passes through different areas and neighborhoods. I'd drive to an access point and walk to the next access point or two, perhaps a mile away. Then I'd walk back. The next time I'd go, I'd drive to the new access point and go further on. Because I was walking to and from my car, while I trekked 30 miles of trail, I had actually walked over sixty miles. Sometimes I invited friends to come along. My husband sometimes joined me. Even when I walked alone, it often felt like a prosocial activity. Others walking the trail often smiled or commented in passing, and more than once, I found myself engaged in a conversation with a total stranger.

At least before the pandemic, shopping malls would open their doors before the stores opened. People who wanted to walk without being subjected to the weather would walk around the mall. Often, they would make and meet friends. Most but not all were seniors, and after a nice walk, you'd see groups of them sitting around the food court with cups of coffee chatting away.

After I had back surgery with more than six months of recovery time, I took a job bagging groceries at a local supermarket just to move my body. The money wasn't important, but the movement was. And in many ways, the job was fun because it wasn't important to me. After all, I have a master's degree. Bagging groceries was never a career option. I did a good job, of course, and the job never caused me stress. Certainly, some of my neighbors who saw me working at the end of the check-out line might have wondered if I had fallen on hard times. But I didn't care. It was fun, and I could quit whenever I wanted.

You'll find something and until you do, walk more and more.

Chapter 12:
The Appointment

———— ⚜ ————

Six months after my doctor tried to prescribe a third medication for my diabetes, the day of my next appointment arrived. I had never called him back, and I expected to be in for a lecture. Given my progress, though, I hoped he would not scold me too much.

In the meantime, I had watched my blood sugar levels decline, especially after my natural fast, which I didn't often finish until lunchtime. While I continued to test my blood when I woke up, I began to psychologically disregard the reading. Having learned about the dawn phenomenon, I considered those readings to be more an indication of my insulin resistance than a true fasting blood glucose reading. But I'm not too sure about that notion.

Prior to this appointment, I had always gone for blood work as soon as the lab opened because I wanted to eat breakfast right after they took my blood. Back then, I thought 10 or 12 hours of fasting was difficult! This time, I went in the late morning. That would be a more accurate reading anyway, and I was in no hurry to eat. I had rarely eaten breakfast in the last three or four months and decided it would be best to go to the lab later in the day, even if it meant spending more time in a crowded waiting room. I was hedging my bets.

Of course, we went out to lunch after! It was a minor celebration, and I felt a kind of relief after the phlebotomist took my blood. It felt like I was playing poker, and I had just gone all in. Everything I had gone through over the last six months was riding on that labwork.

I wasn't really concerned about the fasting blood glucose measurement. I expected it to be in the 90s or, at the highest, the low 100s, as it had been for weeks. I wondered about the A1c. I had tried to calculate an A1c on my own using a formula I had found online but didn't believe the results of my calculations to be accurate as I had based them only on the first preprandial (before eating) readings of the day. The readings after eating were always higher. Although the possibility seemed promising, I knew a hand calculation was inaccurate.

I should backtrack a bit further so you can better understand my confidence. It went well beyond fasting glucose measurements.

A couple of weeks after my low blood sugar episode, it very nearly happened again. A test before a meal read in the attention-getting 70s. I stopped taking the sulfonylurea entirely. A week after that, I decided to drop the metformin as well. Metformin inhibits gluconeogenesis, that is, the conversion of glycogen to glucose, and in my mind, I wanted gluconeogenesis to occur. Not being a doctor or scientist, I didn't think I could get into ketosis while taking metformin. Apparently, some people can enter ketosis on metformin, but I don't think it's common. In any case, I didn't enter ketosis until after I stopped taking the medication, so I'll personally never know.

I wanted to see what my body would do. After stopping those medications, there seemed to be slightly higher numbers, but I never saw a blood glucose reading high enough to worry me after that. By the time I went for my blood work, I hadn't taken any diabetes medications for more than three months.

Before beginning my journey, someone had mentioned to me that if my postprandial reading was 140 or less, I was alright. While on my program, one of the biohacking keto educators I watched on YouTube said that a true postprandial *spike* was 30 points or more above a preprandial reading. My postprandial readings were sometimes above 140 and sometimes represented a real spike even if lower than 140. I figured if they were lower than 140, I was good. If they went above that number, I'd wait to eat until the readings dropped to lower than 110, usually closer to 100. If I spiked more than 30 points, I reconsidered what I had eaten that might have caused the spike. Had I eaten anything unusual? Were there hidden carbs somewhere? Had I eaten more than usual?

I expected that I was still insulin resistant, but my only indication was that dawn phenomenon reading, and six months into my journey, they still seemed erratic. I later determined that reading first thing in the morning was uninformative and just stopped testing at that time. I'd save a finger or two. I also stopped testing right before bed unless my postprandial reading for my last meal were unexpectedly high. My highest postprandial spike usually occurred an hour after eating, so to save fingers, I didn't bother with the 30-minute or 2-hour readings unless the 1-hour reading was exceptionally high.

I had also gone beyond the natural fast of 16 to 18 hours. Several times a week, I began fasting for longer periods of time. I discussed that process in detail in a previous chapter. By the time my appointment came, I was doing longer fasts of 24 to 36 hours, 2 or 3 times a week, with a sprinkling of longer fasts of up to 75 hours every few weeks.

Back to the appointment. After the assistant took my vitals, congratulating me on the weight I had lost, I sat nervously in the room waiting for my doctor. I don't know what my doctor thinks I might be doing in that examination room, but he always knocks and then, after a slight pause, enters with a smile. The smile is either well-practiced or genuine. It doesn't matter. He is a nice and genial guy. He is younger than I am, perhaps in his mid-40s or a very good-looking-for-his-age early 50s. His hair has begun to go gray at the temples, and he seems reasonably fit though middle-aged spread has taken hold.

As he sat down at his computer, I started to apologize for not getting back to him about that third medication. He held up his hand to stop my rambling while reading the computer screen. I didn't take it as rude. After all, he is a very pleasant fellow, and I wouldn't have expected him to memorize my results before our appointment. After a moment, he turned to look at me. He didn't say anything. He didn't ask me any questions. He just waited, giving me a chance to spill my guts. I'm familiar with that trick, but I spilled anyway. My rambling ended with ". . . and I haven't taken my diabetes medications for three months," handing him my spreadsheet, which he barely glanced at.

With a slight shrugging gesture, all he said was, "The numbers don't lie."

That's it? The numbers don't lie? No questions, no congratulations, no high-five. I don't know what I really expected or even what I had been hoping for, but it wasn't that. I was nonplussed. That statement was almost dismissive, but I wouldn't believe that about him. I figured he was baffled and likely skeptical. He didn't display much curiosity. He seemed a little put out that I had stopped taking my meds, but then, "the numbers don't lie," do they? I had the feeling that all my rambling about reducing carbohydrates and intermittent fasting was so much noise to him and that he guessed that by our next meeting, I'd be back on those meds because my remission wouldn't last.

Of course, you must be curious about my results. If I remember properly, my fasting blood glucose reading was in the upper 80s. I expected and hoped for the 90s, and I remember being pleased and perhaps relieved by the result. My A1c was 5.4. I'll never forget that! Given that my previous A1c was near 10, prompting my doctor to want to add that third medication to my regime, one might think that a reading of 5.4 warranted at least congratulations from the doctor. A result of 5.4 is not even prediabetic!

What bothered me the most about that encounter was my doctor's lack of curiosity or perhaps his overriding skepticism. As a scientist, shouldn't he want to know what I had done, or was it the mere fact that I hadn't consulted him that perhaps offended him?

It has been nearly three years since that appointment, and my A1c has never been above 5.4. Two years into my journey, I convinced my doctor to prescribe an insulin resistance test. The result indicated that I was insulin sensitive. Though I had met with my doctor every six months, each time telling him about my process, he displayed little curiosity until he saw the insulin resistance result. He always lets me talk. That time, he seemed to listen. He asked a few skeptical questions, but I could never really tell if he was interested or simply being polite. I pointed him in the direction of two online communities, *Low-Carb USA* and *Low-Carb Down Under*. These communities focus on metabolic science and cater mostly to the medical community and people like me who want to learn from them.

I don't know if he followed through. I even gave him a copy of my first book, *The Hypnofasting Program Guide: A Practical Plan to Lose Weight and Control Type 2 Diabetes*. I hope he read it. He's never mentioned it. Perhaps I'll ask him on our next visit.

During one of our appointments, I asked him when he

would remove the diabetes mellitus diagnosis from my file. The question disconcerted him, and he confessed that he didn't even know if it were possible to do that.

I pushed. "Well, could you look into it?" I think that pissed him off a bit.

"I'll consider it when you can eat like me."

Then it was my turn to feel pissed off. There were lots of things I would have liked to have said, but I held my tongue. I wanted to say that I had no idea how he ate and the odds against me ever following those standard dietary guidelines again were astronomical. I also wanted to say that it was the advice of the nutritionist and those standard dietary guidelines that made my diabetes progressively worse. Indeed, it had likely caused the diabetes to begin with. I held my tongue because what I really wanted to say was that he had taken an oath to do no harm, and I felt like the treatment and the advice I had been given, the standard advice, had certainly harmed me. As far as I am concerned, his approval is neither required nor desired. After all, the numbers don't lie.

I don't really blame him or the nutritionist. He and both of the nutritionists I consulted honestly believed they were doing the right thing and giving me the best advice. But I ask myself, how many people have to die from symptomatic conditions of metabolic disease before the standard advice changes? The system clings to the bad science of Ancel Keys and seems incapable of admitting he was wrong.

An agency trying to get those standard recommendations to change is the Nutrition Coalition, founded by Nina

Teicholz.

Three years in, I've stopped the frequent testing, of course. I don't need it. I do test my blood if I think I've eaten something out of the ordinary, but it's more out of curiosity than concern. I was a good diabetic, and I'm pretty good at keeping up the deleting diabetes lifestyle I've developed.

When I visited my godmother after a long Covid separation, she prepared a traditional Italian-American Sunday dinner, pasta, meatballs, salad, and because it was a special occasion, chocolate cake. I ate reasonable portions of everything, not wanting to underappreciate her effort. My blood glucose spiked because I wasn't used to eating that many carbohydrates. Hell, even the meatballs are half bread crumbs! It was an expected spike, so I didn't worry about it.

I had wondered if eating that meal would trigger old carb cravings for pasta and cake. Happily, it did not. Some months later, when we were invited to dine at a friend's house, he prepared a potato soup. I enjoyed a moderate portion without concern for my blood sugar nor the potential for rejuvenated cravings. It was delicious soup, and I am in control of what I eat.

One of the most liberating feelings is that if I happen to be somewhere, a restaurant perhaps, where there is nothing I think worth eating, I can easily choose to simply not eat until later, even days later, if need be. Practicing therapeutic intermittent fasting comes in handy.

All that being said, I am still careful about what I eat. If you know anyone who has ever been arrested, you might know that the fingerprints and the charge for which they were arrested remain on file forever, even if they were acquitted of the crime or the conviction was expunged. They will spend the rest of their lives marked by that arrest in some way. I suppose that it will be the same for the diagnosis of diabetes mellitus for me. My doctor never followed up on removing the diagnosis, and it remains on my medical record. Until things change, we—you and I—know the truth. I am not diabetic. Diabetes has been deleted from my life.

Like in a computer, I don't know if the diabetes file has been overwritten in a permanent way. Perhaps I'll never know. It's no longer important. The file, I suppose, can be rewritten easily enough by just doing what I did before. If I go back to eating all those carbs and grazing all day, I'll be diabetic again because that was how I became diabetic in the first place. I don't need medications. My body is functioning well. In fact, I am healthier now, at 61 years old, than I have been in my adult life. That is enough for me.

Chapter 13:
Barriers, Obstacles, and the Challenge

---◦❦◦---

D riving across the country twice in my life, I have looked at the landscape and wondered how early settlers got their wagon trains through the vast expanses of desert and the steep mountains. I suppose if they saw that terrain as a true barrier, they just might have given up. I sincerely wonder how many just turned back, stopped somewhere along the road where they thought they might survive, or just died along the way.

No doubt, some of the people who were daunted by the trip actually did stop or even turned back. They likely warned the people who still dreamed of seeing the sun set over the Pacific Ocean of the perils of their journey. Still, they came—wagon trains of them, one after another.

A real barrier can't be conquered or destroyed. A barrier doesn't slow down progress; it stops it. The only way to address a true barrier is to make peace with its existence and live with it.

Thankfully, most barriers are really just obstacles, hurdles in the road that we perceive as barriers. Once we stop moaning and complaining about their existence and begin examining them, studying them, and plotting against them, we see that most barriers are just obstacles we haven't encountered before.

At the beginning of this book, I told you about the boy named Jerrod, who inspiredly found his way across a set of monkey bars by crawling on top of them rather than trying to swing from rung to rung. When he first saw those monkey bars, he saw a barrier. He had tried many times to approach them the normal, expected way and always failed. When he saw the monkey bars as part of his scouting obstacle course, he was intimidated by them. As he approached them, however, his mind decided to see the challenge in a different light. As he approached them, the inner voice that had once resigned itself to believing he couldn't manage the task changed focus. He wondered how he might go about the task differently. In effect, that inner voice stopped moaning, *I can't, I can't* and started asking, *How can I? How can I?* Although approaching the obstacle in a new way required some risk, those monkey bars magically transformed from a barrier to merely an obstacle, little more than a hurdle in a race, and he successfully navigated the apparatus.

I imagine, to a great extent, that's how European settlers

made it to the Pacific coast. No doubt there were discouragements and new challenges along the way, but they ultimately got to see the sun set over the ocean for their reward.

For me, diabetes had been a barrier until I decided I was willing to take the risk of looking at it differently. If I were going to have to live with it, I would approach it with understanding and knowledge rather than ignorance and fear. Somewhere inside myself, I found the courage to stand up to the diabetes bully and vow to go down fighting.

In the process of my courage, mixed with a little desperation, type 2 diabetes became merely an obstacle for me. It was no longer a barrier. Like Jerrod, I thought I could see my way through it. It was at least *possible*. It took a big risk, but it seemed to me a risk worth taking. Others had claimed victory but believing them was a choice. There had been far too many testimonials about superfoods and miracle cures for me to approach my journey without some skepticism. I chose to believe it was possible. I chose to begin the journey. And like those early European settlers, I had no idea really what it would take to reach my destination.

Now I'm going to be a bit tough on you. Please forgive me but I have to do it.

Now *you* have a choice. Will you set out on the journey? Or, will you just stay where you are and live as best you can? Is type 2 diabetes a barrier or an obstacle for you? If it is a barrier, I'm afraid you are stuck. Take your medications, follow the traditional advice and live with your barrier. But at least be the best type 2 diabetic you can be. Understand your body and at least make better decisions. You would be choosing to live with that looming doom of rotting from the inside out, mostly because you believe you can't live without cake. And you can't have your cake and eat it too.

Reconcile yourself to the diabetes prognosis of a chronic and progressive disease. Enjoy your milkshakes, cakes, cookies, french fries, and console yourself with diet soda pop. Enjoy the consolation they give you and eventually fill your body with injected insulin to prolong your life and pack on the pounds. Live the best you can and make the most out of your life. Maybe you're right. Maybe you can't do it.

If that is you, I respect your decision and sincerely wish you well. You are finished reading this book. I thank you for your time, and I hope you enjoyed my story. I wish you the best of luck.

On the other hand, if you are brave enough to take that first step, commit to learning about your body, and stand up to the challenges with the attitude of young Jerrod, I've got a gift for you. Read on.

Chapter 14:
Take a Moment and Breathe

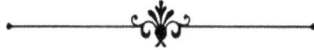

Congratulations on the most difficult step, that first step toward taking ownership and responsibility for your own health, wellness, and happiness. Pat yourself on the back. You deserve it.

Two elements in addition to the dietary regime will play a large role in your success, your ability to relax and, if necessary, improve your sleep. Finding a local clinical hypnotist can be of great help with both relaxing and sleeping. You can also learn to relax more using apps on your phone, joining a meditation group, practicing tai chi, yoga, and even attending prayer services.

Let's try a simple relaxation technique now. Put yourself now in a comfortable, relaxed position. Close your eyes and become aware of your body. Just scan your body from top to bottom, hand to hand, foot to foot, head to toe. Look for areas that feel tense, anxious, impatient. Imagine the muscles, tissues, tendons, and even the cells in those areas beginning to relax, go limp. Imagine it in any way you can. If you feel an itch, try observing it rather than scratching it. Notice any feelings, sensations, or emotions you are having and just observe them, almost as if you are watching someone else experience them.

Now focus your attention on your breath. Just notice breathing in and out. Notice that some breaths are longer or deeper than others. As you relax, notice how your breath becomes more rhythmic, more calm. Notice how when you breathe out, your body actually relaxes a bit more each time.

When you're in that state of relaxation, and you feel you are ready, take a moment and consider the decision you have just made. Tell yourself you can and will do whatever it will take. Don't try to figure out what it will take. Just know that you don't have to cross any bridges or make any other decisions until you come to them, and when you come to them, you'll be ready. You may not be ready for them now, but you don't need to be. Just accept that if there is rough terrain ahead, you'll be ready for it and up to the task. After all, you've made it this far. Take a few more deep breaths and open your eyes.

You've just hypnotized yourself and told your unconscious mind to not be afraid, to not needlessly worry. You will learn. You will see through the bravado of the bully, and you will run the bully off.

I want to tell you another story here. The story belongs to my old friend Tom. He told it at a reunion of school friends. I'll do my best to relay it faithfully here. Tom was picking up one of his nephews from school. Bennie was seven years old and quite tall for his age, a full head above every other kid in his class. Through the rear-view mirror, Tom noticed that Bennie seemed preoccupied. He was munching apple slices, but his mind was somewhere else, and the expression on his face was a worried one.

"What's the matter, Bennie?" Tom asked.

"Nuthin," Bennie mumbled.

After repeating that cryptic conversation a couple of times, my friend pulled over and climbed into the back seat with his nephew.

"Dude, I can tell something is on your mind. Maybe I can help."

Shrugging his shoulders, Bennie admitted he was being bullied because of his height. One boy was instigating the bullying, but others joined in.

When we were growing up, our school district was rather rough. Fistfighting wasn't an uncommon way of resolving conflict.

"He picks on you, and you are bigger than he is?" Tom was incredulous.

Bennie nodded.

"Did you tell the teacher?"

Shaking his head, Bennie said, "She can hear him. Everybody does."

Hearing this, Tom was angered. "I'll tell you how to stop him. The next time he does that, don't run away. Don't yell at him. Just walk up to him very slowly, get real close, so you are looking down at him, and only he can hear you. Then whisper, 'You need to stop. You need to leave me alone. If you don't stop, I am going to beat you up.'"

"We're not allowed to fight."

"You won't have to. I promise."

Tom recounted that he got a call from his sister the next day.

"What did you tell my son?"

"What do you mean? About what?"

"I'm in the principal's office with Bennie and his teacher. They say he threatened another boy, and all Bennie will say is that he did what Uncle Tom told him to do. What did you tell him to do?"

Tom told her about the conversation, and as she tells it, that is Bennie's mother, Tom's sister, who grew up in that same neighborhood, looking directly at the teacher, she said, "You've seen how that boy teases my son, and you've let it happen. If you won't protect my son from a bully, he'll do it himself." Then to her son, "Bennie, if he does it again, kick his ass. You have my permission. Now, let's go home."

At the recounting of this story, we were all laughing.

Given our experience growing up, we all connected with this story. It happened long enough ago that Bennie doesn't even remember it. He is now six-foot-five and plays college football. Nobody in their right mind would try to bully him now.

The story, however, still resonates with me. I don't really want kids to resort to violence to solve problems. Many schools also have anti-bullying policies but how effective they are is open to interpretation. On the other hand, we who have been diagnosed with diabetes live in a world where we are blamed, literally bullied, for being obese and even for being diabetic. We are told it is our fault because we lack self-control, discipline, and willpower. And we take it because we ourselves believe it.

I almost called this book *Kicking Diabetes' Ass*, but I like *Deleting Diabetes* better. Still, I wanted to tell Bennie's story because it works. What I hope you see is that just as Bennie was bigger than the bully, you are bigger than type 2 diabetes, and it's time to take a stand.

When those westward-bound settlers set out on their journey, they never thought of turning back. Neither did they plan to fail. They sold most of their possessions, invested in a covered wagon, and said goodbye to family, friends, and virtually everything they knew, most likely for the rest of their lives, in hopes of a better life with sunsets over the ocean.

As you set out on your own journey, know you will make mistakes. See them as opportunities to learn and adjust your plan accordingly. Resolve to test your blood glucose frequently enough to protect yourself because low blood sugar is a real danger. Determine to understand the medications you are taking. If you don't understand what you are reading, ask your doctor to explain it to you. Commit to sitting through educational videos, reading books, and learning to sift through all the information available to you so that you can decide what is best for you, all the while knowing that what you want to hear may not always be the best.

Abandon the notion of calories, exercise, and diets as temporary measures and embrace a lifestyle change that no longer accommodates type 2 diabetes. Know that you will be uncomfortable and that there will be moments of discouragement and doubt. It can't possibly work out the exact way you expect it to because nothing ever does.

Consult your doctor. If your doctors don't support your decision to reduce carbs and employ intermittent fasting, ask why and ask for the science behind their reasoning. They won't like it, but they should respect your request. If the thought of asking your doctor for their reasoning scares you, first read Ken Berry's book, *Lies My Doctor Told Me*. In fact, bring a copy of it with you as a gift for your doctor.

If your doctor continues to oppose your decision and won't explain why, I suggest you get a second opinion, preferably from a low-carb or ketogenic doctor. They might be hard to find, but I'm certain that some of them at least work online, and a second opinion is well worth paying for out of pocket if your insurance won't cover it.

I'm not suggesting you leave your physician. They know your particular situation better than anyone else. After all, they have your file in front of them and may have been treating you for years. But they may also be relying solely on the information they got in medical school many years ago.

One of the biggest reasons your doctor might not endorse your journey is fear that what happened to Noakes might happen to them. Another is simply they are so unfamiliar with the process that it frightens them to go outside the norm.

If you go it alone as I did, commit to educating your doctor about the process, but the risk is then yours. Look for help. While there may be misinformation out there, low-carb, ketogenic, and intermittent fasting communities can be a source of encouragement and information. Just don't take things at face value. Investigate for yourself.

A new lifestyle includes many changes and can be difficult to navigate. Working with a hypnotist that understands metabolic science can be a great help. Learn about self-hypnosis or meditation to help you along the way. Richard Nongard's book *The Seven Most Effective Methods of Self-Hypnosis* is a good place to start.

Hypnosis may seem odd to you, but hypnosis helps us break old thoughts and behavior patterns. On my most recent visit to my doctor, he asked, "But what does hypnosis have to do with this process?"

"Doc, nobody wants to cut carbs. Nobody wants to fast. That is what hypnosis contributes to this process."

You may not need the help. Lots of people do this process all on their own. If that is you, terrific!

Chapter 15:
A Little Something for the Trip

I can't possibly fully prepare you for your journey in the context of a book. Indeed, that is why all along, I've encouraged you to investigate, learn and grow to understand your own body, its needs, and functions as best you can. The following sections of this chapter address a few of the issues you may encounter on your journey. Most of them are fairly common. If you escape one or more of them, all the better.

Hunger

Most people don't realize that hunger actually happens in their heads. I'm not suggesting that hunger is a figment of the imagination, but all sensations are processed through the brain. Sometimes the triggers of feelings of hunger actually start in the brain. You may feel hungry when walking past a restaurant, at the smell of some delicious food, or while walking through a grocery store. The hunger you feel is not an honest need for nutrition but a response to something completely unrelated to your body's need for food.

Anyone who doesn't eat when they normally eat will feel hungry. If you are used to eating dinner at six in the evening, and you're meeting friends for dinner at 7:30, you'll feel hungry until dinner is served. It's just your internal biological clock telling you that you forgot to eat when you normally eat.

We often associate tummy rumbling with hunger; the truth is, those gurgling sounds have nothing to do with your need for nourishment but are the processing of food you've already eaten through your intestines.

If we have habitually responded to boredom, emotions, or stress by eating something, we'll feel hungry when those feelings are present. It's not real hunger but more likely a desire not to face up to those emotions or stressors. We'll talk more about emotional eating a bit later but for now, know that emotions and stress are not real hunger.

When blood glucose drops, the automatic function of the brain and body may trigger feelings of hunger because the body is experiencing change, even if blood glucose levels are high. It is the breaking away from the normal patterns that cause the hunger. We've been trained to graze, to snack all day. We are bound to feel hungry while breaking that pattern.

You'll find it helpful to examine the possibilities of why you are feeling hungry when hunger pangs surface. You may realize that most often, those feelings have nothing to do with *needing* to eat. Dare I say, in Western society, most of us have never really ever experienced an actual *need* to eat. Even what some people call a hunger headache is more likely due to stress than an empty tummy.

When we feel hungry, it's best not to ruminate over food or what we might possibly eat because to the body, that signals a plan to eat. You may actually be stimulating insulin simply by opening the fridge and looking to see what you might eat. The insulin will reduce your blood glucose levels and make you feel more hungry instead of simply peckish.

By planning when and what you will eat, you begin to take control of your hunger, and you teach your body to recognize new signals for eating. When you feel hungry at other times, observe it. Stop, look at it and observe it as a curiosity. Don't judge it. Don't flee from it. Don't try to reward it with a snack. Just observe it, remind yourself when and what you plan to eat, and tell yourself to wait, so you don't spoil your meal. Then let the hunger go, and it will go away. Say to yourself, *I'll eat my dinner sometime after six this evening.*

When you eat, do it mindfully. Avoid watching television or reading a book, even this one. When we pay attention to our food, we will no longer mindlessly shovel what's on our plate into our mouths. Take your time, focus and taste each bite. Note the texture and flavor as you bite and chew. When you swallow, wait for a few seconds before taking the next bite.

Give the food time to reach your stomach.

Halfway through the meal, stop and examine yourself for feelings of hunger. If you no longer feel hungry, you are satisfied. That means you are done eating until the next meal. Take the rest of your plate, save it for another meal or scrape it into the trash. Eating food when you are not feeling hungry is as much a waste of food as throwing it out. The next time around, take smaller portions. You can always have seconds if you still feel hungry. Eat only until you are satisfied, not full, not overfull, not bloated.

Cravings & Emotional Eating

Cravings are never satisfied by eating what you crave. No one *needs* a donut without then thinking they need another one and another until they've made themselves sick with sugar or guilt. You aren't an animal craving some nutrient hidden in a donut.

No doubt, you will crave carbohydrates as you reduce their role in your eating plan. It's natural. Expect it, but it eventually diminishes and goes away. It just takes time for your body to adjust to different macronutrient ratios.

A craving is a distraction and nothing more. This is why one chip, cookie, or donut is never enough. Usually, cravings distract from something unpleasant, stress, confrontation, guilt, fear, or any myriad of unpleasantries that come with living a normal human life. If you are experiencing cravings, take a moment to check what is prompting the craving and acknowledge that the craving will not be satisfied unless the source of the craving is addressed.

If this sounds like emotional eating, you're absolutely right. Emotional eaters may try to reward themselves for good behavior. *I've been so good. I deserve a piece of cake.* Emotional eaters may feel like compensating themselves for suffering. *I've had a bad day. I deserve a piece of cake.* They may even be punishing themselves for some failure. *Well, I messed up. I might as well eat the whole cake.*

Just like you do with hunger, stop and look for the source or trigger of the craving. If it's stress or anxiety, you need to relax. Do some breathing exercises. If you are bored, a major source of cravings, you need something to do, not something to eat. If you need comfort, ask for a hug, hug yourself or your teddy bear.

Perhaps your mother gave you cookies to stop you bawling like a baby. You learned that cookies happen when you cry, so you want a cookie when you feel like crying. Instead of eating the cookie, have a good cry.

If you find emotional eating to be a huge problem, if in your mind it is a barrier, get some help. I work with emotional eaters all the time. Most emotional eating does not approach the level of a diagnosable eating disorder. Sometimes an eating disorder therapist will refer clients to me for additional help.

Picky Eaters, Veggie Haters, and Mageirocophobics

I've always had an adventurous palate and have been willing to try new foods. That doesn't mean I have liked everything that I've eaten. The first time I tried caviar, I spit it out into a napkin. While in Japan, a friend bought me a huge snail from a street vendor in Kobe. Though the taste was unfamiliar, that is not why

I didn't like it. I didn't like the pungent smell and the flavor that coated my mouth after tasting it.

Note that when I determine I don't like something, I have a specific reason or quality of the food that didn't appeal to me. Just saying I don't like something isn't good enough. I'll explain why that is true a bit later.

Consider my willingness to try those foods. Caviar sounded exotic and something I imagined rich people eat. I have never been rich, so caviar came with a mystique. The snail had neither of those qualities, but I didn't know that I didn't like it until I tried it. The thought of eating snails was initially unappealing, but it was worth giving it a try. I might just like food that initially is unfamiliar.

When you think about what fills the American plate, most of it is actually unappealing to look at. We have somehow convinced ourselves as a society that beige and brown food is appealing. When we were kids, bright colors attracted us, and I suppose that as long as those bright colors were either sweet or sour, we liked them. As we grew into adults, beiges and browns seem to have taken over. The color range of burgers, fries, onion rings, and even pizza is almost monotone. When did brown and beige become appetizing? Perhaps our bodies are so starved for fat we'll eat anything, even fried candy bars, just to get some.

A child who is a picky eater is a bit beyond my experience. I do work with some children, but they have to really want the change. If they don't want the change, we are likely to be unsuccessful, and the parents will be wasting their money. Sometimes kids say they want to change to please their parents, but when push comes to shove, they don't have the necessary followthrough. That being said, there are many great hypnotists who work with children. It's just not my specialty.

I have seen children who have learned how to manipulate their parents into giving them the foods they want. Parents want to see their children grow up healthy and not suffer, but often, that urge, the same one that causes them to attempt to shove food into their infant's mouth, causes them to compromise.

When parents ask me to hypnotize their children to like more foods, I take the time to consult with them. Not always, but often, the problem is that a kid knows if they wait long enough, they will get what they want just because their parents are so desperate to get them to eat. To those parents, I explain that hunger really is the best sauce. If the child doesn't want to eat what the family is eating for dinner, they get to wait until breakfast. If breakfast isn't to their liking, they have to wait until lunch.

School lunches are a problem because they are generally unhealthy meals and the choices for fast food in many schools are a real minefield for most kids. I don't have kids, and I don't know how to handle this problem other than packing a brown bag lunch and monitoring what the child eats, or doesn't eat, in school.

Expanding a teen or adult palate is possible only if they want the change and are willing to work at it. A hypnotist can make liver taste like chocolate or chocolate taste like liver for a while, but that sort of thing doesn't last very long. It is not a solution to the problem. It's an amazing thing to see or experience, but it doesn't solve the issue at hand.

Unfortunately, by the time people call me for help with expanding their palate, that sort of magic is what they are looking for. I can show them a few helpful mind tricks, but I am reluctant to give them a post-hypnotic suggestion of changing chocolate into liver, as might happen in a stage hypnosis show, because I know it won't last. Chocolate does not taste like liver and will find its way back to tasting like chocolate.

I sometimes work with adults on expanding their personal menus, but before I take you through the steps, I want to point out that, in my experience, most adults with a limited palate have very childlike tastes. They tend toward processed and fast foods that kids like. It is important to note that manufactured and fast foods are engineered to achieve a quality of flavor and texture that food researchers call the bliss point. In short, the food item will likely appeal to most people and also has been designed to make people who eat it want more of it. These foods are often target marketed to children who can be persuasive in getting their parents to buy them. Thus, many of my adult clients who wish to expand their palate have always been picky and often manipulative eaters.

If you want to broaden your palate, you have to be willing to open-mindedly try new foods several times before adding them to or cutting them off your menu completely. The process is akin to designing your own bliss point.

When trying new foods, consider each of the following qualities separately and rate your experience of each one. If you don't like a food item, you must be able to say why you don't like it or what about it you don't like. Conversely, if you *do* like it, why or what about that food do you like? It tastes good is not sufficient.

Consider keeping track of your food trials and rate each of the following aspects of the new food on a scale of one to five, one being strongly disliked and five being strongly liked. Consider appearance, smell, temperature, and texture. These aspects of a food are easily changed and can provide a range of experiences. For example, if something doesn't appeal to you cold, it might appeal to you at room temperature or even heated. If something is too crunchy or not crunchy enough, you can change the way you prepare or serve the food. You might not like the texture of chunks of tomato but like tomato sauce. I have a friend who hates celery in salad but likes it cooked in soup. Another eats cucumbers raw while avoiding pickles.

I knew a young man who would only eat veggies pureed in broth, like a creamy soup. If that's the way you need to eat veggies, invest in a stick blender and have at it.

The actual taste of the food is a bit more complicated, but the process is the same. We are going to consider sweetness, tartness, saltiness, and bitterness. If the food is too salty, use less salt the next time around. If it's not salty enough, add a good quality salt. If the food is bland, you have a large variety of things you can do to make it tastier!

I had a roommate from France who was fascinated with my corn popper. Every day, I'd come home from class to see popcorn in the trash. I couldn't figure out why he was throwing away all the popcorn. When I asked him about it, he seemed frustrated. "How do you flavor it? What is the flavor at the movies?"

"Butter and salt."

He had been trying to find the right flavor, and he just hadn't it on butter and salt. I never saw popcorn in the trash again.

A case from my own palate: I don't like cooked peas, but I love them fresh out of the garden, eaten alone or in a salad. I love snow peas in the shell in salad, stir-fried, and in soup. And I don't mind peas if they are pureed in something else, a soup or in a sauce. For me, the problem with peas is the texture of the outer shell and the mushy insides. It's the two textures together that make peas unappealing. The point is that there is only one way I don't like peas but many other ways that I do.

When you determine what aspect does not appeal to you, look for similarities between foods you dislike. Maybe you don't like bitter-tasting foods. Maybe you don't like crunchy foods. Maybe you don't like foods served cold. How might you change these things for your next taste test?

Ask yourself what appeals to you about the food. What associations are you making with the appearance of that food? How might you change the appearance of the food in order to make it more appealing? You can try it again later under different conditions.

Have you noticed I've spent a lot of time talking about vegetables? That is because many picky eaters are most picky about vegetables. Not surprisingly, they all seem to love french fries and mashed potatoes.

Most people who say they don't like vegetables simply

do not know or are unaware of the most creative ways of preparing them. For many years, canned vegetables were our go-to method for preserving them for winter when, in most of the country, fresh produce was locally unavailable.

A person would open a can, dump it into a pot, heat it up, and serve it. The taste of canned vegetables is unmistakable. Frozen veggies were a step up, but as the role of fat in our diet changed, the ways most Americans knew how to cook vegetables became more limited. Butter was seen as bad. Cream sauces, because of the fat, were considered unhealthy. Some of the best ways of enjoying veggies fell by the wayside.

It's no wonder many people don't like vegetables.

When I was a kid, there was a recipe for salad dressing that used warm bacon grease. Poured over the salad, the lettuce would wilt a bit and form a wonderful side dish even if one didn't really consider it a salad. My clients literally brighten when I assure them that they can use real butter, never margarine, and even bacon fat to flavor their veggies.

In the 80s, I went to a literary lunch at the Waldorf Astoria hotel in New York City, celebrating Julia Childs' new cookbook. In her speech, she spoke disparagingly about the trays of raw vegetables served as finger foods at parties, something popular back then. I wish I could quote her directly, but I don't think my memory is up to a verbatim rendition. As I remember it, she said something like, "No butter, no fat, what kind of party is that?" I also noticed she didn't touch the lunch the Waldorf Astoria served us, and I'll bet she lambasted her publisher for being so cheap with the food.

One of the wonderful things about the internet is the ready availability of recipes for unique ways of serving different dishes. All you have to do is go to YouTube and do a search naming a vegetable with the word recipe. Some of them need adapting to be low carb, but that often isn't difficult. Instead of using flour to thicken a sauce, use heavy cream. It's easy.

Of course, following a recipe assumes that a person does not suffer from mageirocophobia, an irrational fear of cooking. The first time I watched a few episodes of the Food Network show *Worst Cooks in America*, I was aghast and shocked at the absurdity of the contestants who had grown up to adulthood without knowing how to fry an egg. How did they survive? What garbage have they been eating? I also noticed that contestants who would say things like, "I'll never be able to do this," got eliminated early.

In my high school, boys took wood shop, and girls took home economics. Sexist, I know, but that was the seventies. Let me make you feel a little better. For several weeks a year, we switched—the boys took home economics, and the girls made stuff out of wood. Sexism still reigned, though. The things boys cooked were things like hotdogs wrapped in crescent rolls that came out of a tube. We made spaghetti using sauce out of a jar. And we burned grilled cheese sandwiches. The only recipe we really followed was one for chocolate chip cookies. We didn't learn how to cook. We learned how to survive until some woman married us and took over for our mothers.

As for me, by the time I was in the fifth grade, I was cooking my own breakfast. I made oatmeal, eggs, and even pancakes. I wielded a bread knife and sliced my mother's homemade bread in even slices without mangling it. I learned to do those things. My father and brother also knew how to do those things within the context of a traditional, first-generation, Italian-American family in which it was considered the woman's job to do those things.

Anyone can learn how to follow a recipe and cook real food. Talent may play a part in finesse or improvisation in the kitchen. But anyone, and I mean anyone, can follow a recipe. If you think you can't cook and you have to depend on restaurants, processed frozen food, or packaged meals, you owe it to yourself and the people you love to take a cooking class. Do it with a friend. Do it with your spouse. Do it with your children and give up that story you are telling yourself that you can't cook. There is no more important skill for survival. And, you just may find out that you've been needlessly depriving yourself of good, real food for years.

Well-meaning opposition

You will encounter situations and people that work against your goals. There will be people who cajole you to eat with them. They will insist you eat everything they have prepared. People who know you are fasting will express concern for you. They will say you are on some fad diet. Even doctors and nutritionists might want to insist on you eating high-carbohydrate food as part of a "balanced diet."

Your relationships with some people will change. If all you do with certain friends is eat out, you will eventually have to find something else to do or accept the label as the healthy one in the group who doesn't eat. There may be situations at certain restaurants where nothing on the menu is worth eating. Your friends will have to either accept your decision not to eat and leave well enough alone, or there will be some sort of confrontation. I've had friends insist we get up from the table and go to a different restaurant despite my protests.

Here are some hints for navigating sticky situations involving well-meaning opposition.

Be judicious about who knows you are fasting. I often tell people I am not hungry, even if I am feeling hungry. It's a white lie, but I'd rather act like I'm not hungry than have to explain to them in tedious detail why I'm not eating. Even the Bible recommends combing your hair and washing your face when you fast (Matthew 6:17). In my mind, that means look normal, smile, be pleasant and nice, and don't stare longingly at other people's food.

My husband accused me of starving myself when I began longer fasts. I stood my ground. "I could make it through seven years of famine," I said, grabbing the rolls of fat on my belly. He still didn't understand, but I couldn't help that. "You're not diabetic," I would say. It didn't sway him. His concern was real, but my not eating made meals more complicated. I'd sit with him at the table and try to have a conversation, but he felt uncomfortable eating in front of me. I started making excuses like I had eaten a late lunch. If you don't like lying, "I've already eaten" technically is not a lie. You have eaten in the past. You don't have to be specific about when.

When you refuse food because you know it's not good for you, do not tell people why. You don't have to point out the unhealthy oils, the amount of carbohydrates, or the added sugar. Doing so will only make you seem pompous or insufferable. A simple "no thank you" should suffice. If it doesn't, and they cajole you, try, "I'm not hungry." If that doesn't work, a slightly more direct but still respectful comment is, "I am allowed to not eat something if I am not hungry" or "I simply don't want to eat it."

At first, if I were in a restaurant with friends, I'd order something and then not eat it. I'd say I had already eaten or make some other excuse. That got expensive, especially if when I got home, my doggie bag went into the trash. Later, I learned how to order things that had better macro ratios. I might order a burger without the bun or a salad and use just lemon wedges, salt, and pepper for dressing. I often make my own dressing and bring it to the restaurant. If I order a bacon and egg breakfast, I don't want the potatoes or the toast, but if that flusters the server, I just don't eat them. There always seems to be someone willing to eat my fries. I don't have to make excuses when they are eating my fries.

Don't criticize or comment on the unhealthy eating habits you see in others. Don't tell them why it's bad for them or why they shouldn't eat it. If they see your change, they may ask, but I have severely diabetic friends who are not the slightest bit interested in what I've done. They are happy for me but are not able to see themselves doing what I have done.

You will encounter situations that frustrate you, baffle you, surprise you and make you laugh, and even make you cry. The toughest part is simply staying focused long enough to truly see evidence of your progress.

Within weeks of beginning my journey, I experienced low blood sugar, but that didn't inspire me. I was alone and afraid. When I decided to cut my medications, I fully expected that I was taking a serious risk. When I started drilling extra holes in my belt, I was encouraged even though I wasn't intent on losing weight. It took a long time for me to notice the downward trajectory of my blood glucose readings.

I read somewhere that the liver rejuvenates completely in three years. In my mind, I committed to that length of effort. It's now three years in, and my blood sugar levels are fine when I test them. My diabetes is still deleted, but I don't know if it has yet been overwritten. I am still a little overweight, and I've got crepey skin hanging on my body. I have more energy and am in better health now, at 61 years old, than I have ever been in my adult life. Though I made many mistakes and had a few false starts, there was one notion from the very beginning that I was right about: The change had to be permanent and, thereby, sustainable. There was nothing temporary about it.

Take your journey one step at a time, and if you overeat carbs in a fit of cloudy-headed weakness or overwrought emotions, don't hate yourself. If you don't finish a fast as you planned, don't see it as a failure but as a learning opportunity. Give yourself credit for having made gains. Gains are never truly lost unless you forsake them completely.

Pat yourself on the back regularly for every step forward, and if there are steps backward, know that you are still ahead because it all adds up. Every step brings you closer and closer to your goal.

About the Author

❧

Joseph Onesta is a clinical hypnosis practitioner in private practice at Mind Power Pittsburgh in Pittsburgh, Pennsylvania. While he is a skillful generalist able to help clients with a wide variety of issues, he specializes in the areas of metabolic disease, anxiety, depression, and sleep difficulties. He sees clients in person in his Pittsburgh office as well as online.

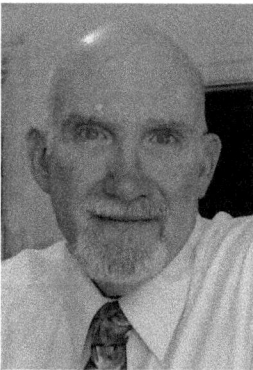

Joseph is the author of two other books, *The Hypnofasting Program Guide: A Practical Plan to Lose Weight and Control Type 2 Diabetes* and *Uneasy Faith: How to Survive Religious Trauma without Sacrificing Spirituality.*

Frequently, Joseph speaks and educates other hypnotists at hypnosis conferences and supervises the clinical practice of new hypnotists. He is available to address groups on the subjects of clinical hypnosis and the role of hypnosis in addressing metabolic disease. He can be reached through his website, www.MindPowerPittsburgh.com.

Suggested Reading or Listening

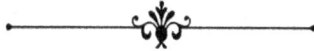

❧

The following books are available in paperback and audio versions. I've provided enough information for you to find the books or the recordings wherever you buy them. What strikes me most about the list is how old many of the titles are. You can get many, if not most, of them from used and discounted booksellers. I don't have an affiliate link; these titles are what I've read and, in most ways, endorse. Of course, you make your own decisions about them. Have a fun and rewarding journey. I did.

Berry, Ken D. *Lies My Doctor Told Me: Medical Myths That Can Harm Your Health.* Las Vegas: Victory Belt Publishing Inc., 2019.

Fung, Jason, and Nina Teicholz. *The Diabetes Code: Prevent and Reverse Type 2 Diabetes Naturally.* Vancouver: Greystone Books, 2018.

Fung, Jason. *The Cancer Code: A Revolutionary Understanding of a Medical Mystery*. London: Thorsons, 2020.

Fung, Jason. *The Obesity Code Unlocking the Secrets of Weight Loss*. Melbourne: Scribe, 2016.

Lierre, Kieth. *Vegetarian Myth Food, Justice, and Sustainability*. Crescent City, CA: Flashpoint Press, 2009.

Noakes, Timothy, and Marika Sboros. *Real Food on Trial: How the Diet Dictators Tried to Destroy a Top Scientist*. United Kingdom: Columbus Publishing, 2019.

Nongard, Richard K. *The Seven Most Effective Methods of Self-Hypnosis: How to Create Rapid Change in Your Health, Wealth, and Habits*. Scottsdale, AZ: Expert Leadership Performance, 2019.

Perlmutter, David. *Brain Maker: The Power of Gut Microbes to Heal and Protect Your Brain - for Life*. London: Yellow Kite, 2017.

Perlmutter, David. *Grain Brain: The Surprising Truth about Wheat, Carbs, and Sugar - Your Brain's Silent*. Hodder & Stoughton Ltd., 2014.

Taubes, Gary. *Good Calories Bad Calories*. Gary A. Knopf, 2007.

Taubes, Gary. *The Case against Sugar*. London: Portobello, 2018.

Taubes, Gary. *Why We Get Fat: And What We Can Do About It.* New York: Alfred A. Knopf, 2011.

Teicholz, Nina. *The Big Fat Surprise: Why Butter, Meat, and Cheese Belong in a Healthy Diet.* New York: Simon & Schuster Paperbacks, 2015.

www.ingramcontent.com/pod-product-compliance
Lightning Source LLC
Chambersburg PA
CBHW050724030426
42336CB00012B/1409